C. Circulation
- If pulse absent, start ECC.
- Depress the lower part of sternum 1½ to 2 inches, approximately 2 inches above xiphoid process.
- The basic steps are determine consciousness, extend airway, give four quick ventilations, check carotid pulse, and start compression-ventilation cycle.

- *Single-person rescue:* give 15 compressions (11 seconds and 2 ventilations (4 seconds). Repeat cycle at 15:2 ratio, rate of 80 compressions per minute. Recheck pulse in 1 minute.

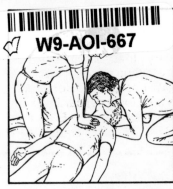

- *Two-person rescue:* give 5 compressions (1 per second) and 1 ventilation on fifth upstroke. Repeat cycle at 5:1 ratio, rate of 60 compressions per minute. Recheck pulse in 1 minute and when switching positions.

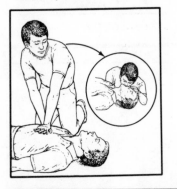

Single-person rescue

Reminders:
Call 911 for Emergency Medical Service. Continue CPR until the ambulance arrives. Recheck pulse whenever second rescuer arrives at the scene. The two-person rescue is always more effective than a single-person rescue.

Refer to Chapter 4 for detailed instructions in CPR.

The Common Sense Medical Guide and Outdoor Reference

The Common Sense Medical Guide and Outdoor Reference

Newell D. Breyfogle

University of California, Santa Barbara

Medical Advisors
Sherman C. Meschter, M.D.
John A. Reyburn, Jr., M.D.

Illustrated by
Allan Parker

McGRAW-HILL BOOK COMPANY
New York   St. Louis   San Francisco   Auckland   Bogotá
Guatemala   Hamburg   Johannesburg   Lisbon   London
Madrid   Mexico   Montreal   New Delhi   Panama   Paris
San Juan   São Paulo   Singapore   Sidney   Tokyo   Toronto

THE COMMON SENSE MEDICAL GUIDE AND OUTDOOR REFERENCE

Copyright © 1981 by McGraw-Hill, Inc. All rights reserved. Printed in the United States of America. No part of this publication may be reproduced, stored in a retrieval system, or transmitted, in any form or by any means, electronic, mechanical, photocopying, recording, or otherwise, without the prior written permission of the publisher.

This book was set in Century Schoolbook by Monotype Composition Company, Inc. The editors were Robert P. McGraw and Moira Lerner; the designer was Merrill Haber; the production supervisor was Jeanne Skahan.

The photographs preceding Parts 1 and 2 and the appendixes were done by Reginald Wickham.

Library of Congress Cataloging in Publication Data

Breyfogle, Newell D
    The common sense medical guide and outdoor reference.

    Bibliography: p.
    Includes index.
    1. Medical emergencies. 2. Outdoor life—Accidents and injuries.
I. Title. [DNLM:
1. Emergencies—Popular works. 2. Recreation—Popular works.
3. Medicine—Popular works.
WB 120 B849c]
RC86.7.B74   616'.025   80-27326
ISBN 0-07-007672-3
ISBN 0-07-007673-1 (pbk.)

This guide is dedicated to all those it may serve

Contents

List of Consultants

Perry P. Amick, M.D.
Associate Physician,
Student Health Service,
College Health Medicine/Pediatrics,
University of California, Santa Barbara

John A. Baumann, M.D.
Director, Student Health Service,
College Health Medicine/Sportsmedicine,
University of California, Santa Barbara

Blaine A. Braniff, M.D.
Internal Medicine/Cardiology,
Santa Barbara Cardiovascular Group

Celia C. Breyfogle, R.N.
Director of Nurses, Student Health Service and
Family Planning Nurse Practitioner,
University of California, Santa Barbara

Florence K. Furukawa, R.Ph.
Senior Pharmacist, Student Health Service,
University of California, Santa Barbara

Herbert A. Grench, Ph.D.
General Manager, Midpeninsula Regional
Open Space District,
Outdoor and Wilderness Education,
Los Altos

Wayne Horodowich, M.A.
Lecturer, Physical Activities,
Outdoor and Wilderness Education,
University of California, Santa Barbara

Sherman C. Meschter, M.D.
Associate Physician, Student Health Service,
College Health Medicine,
University of California, Santa Barbara

Robert J. Offerman, M.D.
Orthopedic Surgery
Orthopedic Group of Santa Barbara

Finlay E. Russell, M.D., Ph.D.
Professor of Neurology, Physiology, and Biology,
University of Southern California;
Director, Laboratory of Neurological Research,
Los Angeles County,
University of Southern California Medical Center

John A. Reyburn, Jr., M.D.
Associate Physician Diplomat, Internal Medicine,
Institute of Environmental Stress and Student
Health Service,
University of California, Santa Barbara

Cindy Sage, M.A.
Lecturer, Environmental Studies,
Outdoor and Wilderness Education,
University of California, Santa Barbara

Orrin Sage, Jr., Ph.D.
Lecturer, Environmental Studies,
Outdoor and Wilderness Education,
University of California, Santa Barbara

Bruce Tegner, B.A.
Lecturer, Outdoor Education,
Outdoor and Wilderness Education,
Ventura College and University of California Extension,
Santa Barbara

Preface

The Common Sense Medical Guide and Outdoor Reference is directed to families, students, boaters, campers, and backpackers to enhance their abilities to prepare for, recognize, and cope with various medical emergencies.

The guide divides naturally into two parts. The first part deals with the commonsense approach to handling medical emergencies. This section is presented in a simple, straightforward manner to assist the nonmedical person in recognizing and treating medical emergencies. Every effort has been made to present currently accepted medical facts in a manner which makes them of practical value. The second part provides a unique feature not commonly found in the usual texts on first aid and emergency medical care. It provides specific information on how to prepare for, how to anticipate, and how to handle many outdoor and wilderness emergencies.

The appendixes provide an added dimension with a special section on cancer; the "Medicine Chest," which lists medications and tells how to take prescription drugs; and an extensive listing of first-aid and emergency kits. An unusual approach is presented in the Glossary, which not only identifies terms but in many cases provides information on how to recognize and treat the problem.

The purpose of this guide is to provide enough information for the reader to feel secure and confident in the management of unexpected circumstances in the home, on the road, or on a short trip into the wilderness. I trust it will effectively serve this purpose.

Acknowledgments

In developing *The Common Sense Medical Guide and Outdoor Reference* I am grateful to a number of individuals who have made significant contributions toward its completion. The medical procedures contained in this guide are based upon current practices and recommendations of individuals from the medical profession.

I am especially indebted to John A. Reyburn, Jr., M.D., and Sherman C. Meschter, M.D., for their advice and the accuracy of the material. With the aid of their watchful eyes and critical analysis, we have provided the nonmedical person with the most accurate and up-to-date medical guide of its kind.

I am appreciative of the many suggestions and contributions of physicians from the University of California Student Health Service and the city of Santa Barbara. My thanks to Drs. Perry P. Amick, John A. Baumann, and Blaine A. Braniff. They graciously gave their time and energy reviewing the manuscript.

My wife Celia's critical suggestions and contribution in writing the section on common medical disorders for women were indeed appreciated.

The advice, comments, and contributions of Orrin Sage, Jr., Ph.D., and Cindy Sage on the "Outdoor Reference" section were invaluable. Their participation in the Emergency and Wilderness Medicine seminars with Finlay E. Russell, M.D., John A. Reyburn, Jr., M.D., John A. Baumann, M.D., Herbert A. Grench, Ph.D., Wayne Horodowich, and Bruce Tegner provided impetus in the development of the guide.

Sincere thanks are due to my daughter Laura for the preliminary editing of the material.

The U.S. Department of Commerce, National Oceanic and Atmospheric Administration, graciously provided many of the photographs.

A very special thanks to the two Pams for their assistance in the preparation of the guide: to Pamela White for typing the manuscript and to Pamela Green for her superb role in editing and shaping the format of the guide into its present form.

Finally, I give profound thanks to the many friends from the medical and outdoor education profession whose ears I have bent in order to gain the most current information available. I am indebted to all of you.

Newell D. Breyfogle

Part 1

Common Sense Medical Guide

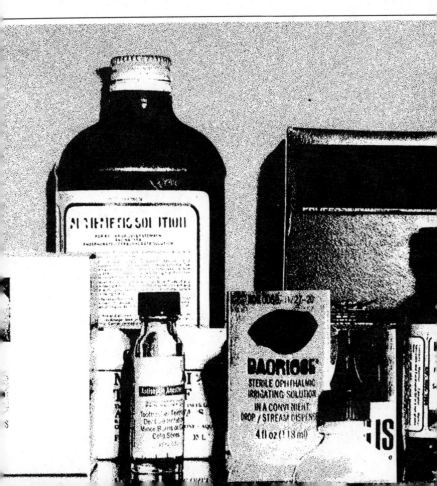

Chapter 1

Introduction to Common Medical Emergencies

Medical emergencies vary from the simple to the complex and from situations in which medical assistance is readily available to those in which it is quite inaccessible. Three basic steps should be taken in dealing with medical emergencies. First of all, one must establish the urgencies involved; second, one must handle and treat the victim; and third, one must obtain proper medical assistance. Immediate attention must be given to victims of an accident or sudden illness until they can receive appropriate professional attention. The length of this care will vary, depending upon the location of the accident or illness and the availability of medical assistance. The farther you are from a community and telephone, the more you will need to develop your ingenuity, skills, and resources if an illness or accident occurs.

The aid you extend to the injured person will affect the victim emotionally as well as physically, so you must deal with the entire situation. It is important to know *what to do*, as well as *what not to do*, in handling emergencies. The proverb "First, do no harm" is the best rule to follow! Fortunately, most accidents or illnesses are not life-and-death situations, and with proper attention, care, and planning can be adequately handled. The care given an accident victim should involve common sense and good judgment.

Of the many medical emergencies one encounters, only a few are really critical or "hurry" cases. This means that prompt, immediate attention must be provided if the victim is to survive. Critical cases include:

- Stoppage of breathing
- Stoppage of the heart (sudden cardiac arrest)
- Severe bleeding

Once successful treatment has been given (airway opened, breathing and/or heartbeat restored, or bleeding controlled), attention should be directed at preventing or minimizing the state of physical shock. Shock may occur shortly after an accident or be delayed for several hours. Supportive measures can reduce its effects. Refer all victims to a medical facility.

Two other very serious but less urgent cases where quick emergency action must be taken are severe poisoning and heatstroke. Specific treatment is discussed later in the guide.

The possibility of serious head, neck, or spinal injury constitutes another grave medical emergency. The victim should be kept very still and transferred by ambulance and qualified personnel to a hospital. In accidents requiring any advanced medical care, the person should be taken directly to a hospital emergency department. If the victim is seriously ill or the symptoms are too severe to endure—the pain is acute, persistent, or recurring—call a physician.

Many minor injuries and illnesses can be adequately treated in the home or the wilderness if proper first aid is administered. Subsequent chapters will provide information for handling these first-aid problems.

Legal Implications

Most states have passed *good samaritan laws* regarding first aid and cardiopulmonary resuscitation (CPR). The general intent of these laws is to ensure that anyone voluntarily assisting an injured person at the scene of an accident is not held responsible for any acts of omission or commission. It is of primary importance that you do nothing that will compound the existing problem by rendering improper treatment. Immunity is not likely to be granted when gross negligence or willful misconduct occurs. The best defense is to give the proper aid, work within your limitations, and seek the necessary medical assistance. Good training programs will assist you in making these all-important decisions. Each individual should know about the Emergency Medical Services (ambulance) available in the community, the company's policy regarding service, and how to call them. Cost of securing an ambulance usually becomes the responsibility of the injured. If you deem an ambulance, helicopter, or other service necessary for the overall safety and health of the injured person, then by all means obtain it. (Check with the local American Red Cross and American Heart Association regarding good samaritan laws in your state.)

Chapter 2
Techniques of Emergency Care

Preventing Medical Emergencies

Many emergencies occur because people do not pay enough attention to their own behavior. These can be prevented if we think, plan, and prepare in our daily lives. In the pages which follow, many general safety tips will be presented, most of them relating to commonsense awareness of potential hazards. These tips include developing good housekeeping practices; proper use and administration of medication; keeping utensils, tools, and sharp objects in their proper places; planning for trips and emergencies; safe driving practices; and perhaps most important, the education of our families in good first-aid practices and procedures. We should all develop a list of potential problems or hazards in our surroundings to aid in the prevention of accidents. Many accidents occur because of carelessness or impetuosity. In order to prevent accidents, one must be willing to develop patience and plan ahead.

It is important to realize that you can have a great deal of control over whether or not you will be involved in a medical emergency. The development of positive, safe attitudes; a greater awareness of potential hazards; and the institution of good safety precautions will ensure a safe environment.

Accidents, nevertheless, will happen. You should plan for such emergencies. It is important to maintain a well-prepared first-aid kit for all situations—the home, the automobile, the boat, or the outdoors.

A family disaster plan should be developed for potential emergencies in the home or community (fire, flood, earthquake, tornado, hurricane, or blizzard). In any general disaster, lives can be saved if people are prepared for emergencies and know what action to take when they occur.

What to Do if You Witness an Accident

In the management of an accident victim, one should have specific guidelines to follow. The extensiveness of one's plan depends on the seriousness of the accident, the location, the number of people involved, and the proximity and availability of medical assistance.

In general, you should observe the following procedures.

- Take a moment to calm yourself and analyze the entire situation—location of accident, potential hazards, and other problems.
- Formulate a plan and carry it out. Work quickly but carefully. Give proper instructions and account for all victims.

- Utilize all assistance. Do not send help off when vitally needed at scene.

- Establish traffic control, directing traffic if necessary. Flares or emergency flashers may be an early priority. *Caution: Do not place flares near spilled gasoline.*

- Summon assistance (911).[1] Obtain proper Emergency Medical Service (ambulance), rescue units (fire department, search and rescue, Coast Guard), police or law enforcement (for traffic and crowd control): include information on the exact number of victims and on the location and nature of accident.

- Treat the most serious injury. Check for critical cases (airway, breathing, circulation, serious bleeding).

- Check for Medic Alert tags [ID tags designating specific medical problems (see Figure 1)]. They come from the Medic Alert Foundation International, Turlock, CA 95380. Engraved bracelets indicate the medical problems. Lifetime membership costs $10.00. Other companies provide a similar service.

- Treat all victims for possible shock (see Chapter 3, "Shock"). Keep victim quiet and lying down, and maintain body temperature.

- Check for other injuries and treat if appropriate (extensive first-aid treatment, i.e., splinting, usually not indicated if Emergency Medical Services en route and hospital nearby).

- Keep all victims lying down and still; do not allow to stand, sit, or walk.

- Give reassurance: be positive and confident in your actions.

---

[1] 911 is an emergency number to be dialed to obtain immediate assistance from the fire department, police, and Emergency Medical Services (EMS). If it is not available in your community, dial 0 (operator) for medical assistance.

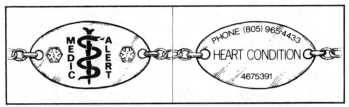

Figure 1   Medic Alert identification bracelet with an example of the reverse side. (Telephone number is a sample only.)

- Do not move any seriously injured persons unless absolutely necessary.
- Do not give fluids to an unconscious or partly unconscious person, or one with head, abdominal, or chest injuries.
- Loosen clothing about the neck and waist; make the victim comfortable.
- If vomiting occurs, turn victims onto their sides to ensure an open airway. (*Caution:* Be aware of possible neck injury.)
- Remove loose dentures and partial plates from the mouth if they obstruct the airway.
- Obtain names and addresses of injured and notify relatives if appropriate. (Usually public officials will perform this task.)
- *Use common sense.*

How to Assist the Victim

Always remember, your attitude is of utmost importance in the management of the victim in a medical emergency. If you can appear composed and relaxed, your attitude will be transmitted to the victim and help to relieve the person's anxieties. Relaxation of the victim may ease respiration, slow any serious bleeding, reduce pain, and decrease the element of shock. You, as the rescuer or the first responder, should initially take several deep breaths to establish your composure. It will give you an opportunity to assess the situation and determine a course of action. Place your hands gently on the victim and speak in soft tones, using his or her name, if you know it, as frequently as possible. This physical and verbal communication will give needed reassurance and encourage the victim's relaxation. *Be positive.* Explain what you are doing and how you can assist during this time of need. The act of appearing composed and in complete control will present the best opportunity for success in a medical emergency.

Examination of Injuries

If an individual is conscious and able to talk, ask the person what happened and where the pain is located. First, you need to recognize the victim's problems as real; next, work within your limitations and abilities in offering advice and/or providing treatment. Priorities in the assessment of suspected problems are airway, breathing, and circulation (breathing impairment, heart involvement, or visible bleeding). If these problems do not exist and medical help is unavailable, examine the person for other injuries, working from head to foot. Usually the injuries at the top of the body are more serious, and the injuries located farther downward, toward the feet, are comparatively less serious. Basic checks that should be made in assessing a person's condition include the following (also refer to Figure 4, later in this chapter):

Head Check for bruises and any area sensitive to touch. Examine the eyes for pupils which are uneven, enlarged, or unresponsive to light. Headaches, disorientation, confusion, or memory problems, coupled with uneven pupil size, may indicate a serious head injury. Individuals may or may not have recall of information; therefore ask victims questions about current conditions and what they were doing when the accident occurred. (The victim's long-term memory is often less impaired than the short-term memory. For example, victims may be able to tell you all the details of their childhood but not have the faintest idea where they are, what they are doing, and how they got there.) Disorientation may be a part of a variety of illnesses and injuries, especially if a high fever is present. If watery fluid or blood is flowing from the nose or ears, it indicates the possibility of a skull fracture.

Neck Check for any pain, stiffness, or soreness in this area. Numbness and tingling sensation in extremities may be present. Without moving the victim, gently run your fingers over the vertebrae to feel for any irregularities. These signs indicate the possibility of neck or cervical spinal injury, and *the person should not be moved*. When in doubt, assume a spinal injury is present.

Chest Gently feel the chest walls for any irregularities. Soreness may indicate bruised or fractured ribs. The coughing up of bright, frothy blood indicates probable injuries to the lungs. Pain or discomfort may be present in breathing. Problems associated with breathing and the heart often follow accidents and should be recognized.

Abdomen If the conscious person complains of pain in the abdomen or if there is tenderness upon palpation, suspect an injury to the liver, spleen, kidneys, or intestine. Firmness of the muscles of the abdomen on the left side may indicate injury to the spleen. An individual passing blood in urine may well have kidney injury.

Arm, Shoulder, Pelvis, and Legs Pain, tenderness, or deformities in these areas indicate possibilities of bruises, sprains, strains, fractures, and/or a dislocation.

Note: The longer it will take medical assistance to reach you, the more complete the examination should be.

Vital Signs and Common Problems

Knowledge of the vital signs in evaluating a person's condition following an accident or sudden illness is important in determining proper medical care.

Consciousness Changes in the state of consciousness may vary from mild confusion to a deep coma as a result of a severe head injury, poisoning, or severe illness. A lapse into a deep state of unconsciousness indicates a need for immediate medical care.

Respiration Normal breathing occurs without pain and effort at a rate of 12 to 16 breaths per minute in adults,

16 to 20 in children, and 20 to 30 in infants. Rapid, shallow, or deep, gasping breaths reflect abnormal breathing patterns. Rapid, shallow breathing is seen in shock and many other conditions. Deep, gasping breaths may indicate airway obstruction or heart and respiratory problems. Absence of breathing indicates respiratory arrest. Stoppage of the heart is one cause of respiratory arrest.

Pulse The normal pulsebeat at rest is 60 to 90 beats per minute in adults and 80 to 100 in infants. The carotid artery in the neck and the radial artery in the wrist are the most common places to feel or palpate the pulse (see Figure 2). The infant's pulse is palpated on the brachial artery, located in the upper inner arm. Rapid, weak pulse is usually a result of shock. Rapid, strong pulse is present in fright. Absence of pulse reflects cessation of the heart.

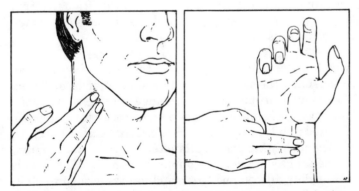

Figure 2 Technique used to palpate (feel) the carotid and radial pulse.

Temperature   The average normal internal temperature of the body is 98.6°F. In emergency care, feel the victim's skin with the back of your hand to estimate temperature. Cool, clammy skin may often reflect shock due to injury and may be present in heat exhaustion. Exposure to cold temperatures may produce cool, dry skin, whereas hot, dry skin may reflect illness or excessive heat exposure, as in heat sroke.

Skin Color   Skin color indicates the presence of circulating blood near the surface of the skin. In deeply pigmented people, color changes can be found in the fingernails and under the tongue. *Red* or flushed condition is associated with a sun- or heatstroke. *White* condition reflects insufficient circulation, as in fainting, shock, or fright. It is also present, *at onset,* in a severe heart attack or a massive stroke. *Blue* condition (lack of O_2 in the blood), referred to as *cyanosis,* may indicate airway obstruction, complete heart failure, drowning, and certain types of gas poisoning. *Yellow* condition, referred to as *jaundice,* is caused by an illness usually associated with liver disease.

Pupil of the Eye   The pupils of the eyes, when normal, are usually the same size, and constrict to light and react together. Unequal pupils or changes in size of the pupils may be the result of a drug or a disease (see Figure 3). Dilated pupils may reflect shock or cardiac arrest (oxygen deficiency). Unequal pupils often indicate head injury. Some drugs will make the pupils very small. If the pupils are widely dilated and fixed, and fail to respond to light,

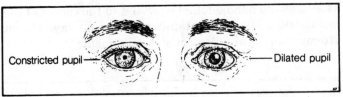

Constricted pupil

Dilated pupil

Figure 3 Normally pupils are equal in size and react together. Pupils may be unequal, dilated, or constricted for various reasons.

death may be imminent. *Note:* Contact lenses make pupils appear larger than normal.

Pain Usually occurs at the site of injury or illness. Pain may be sharp, dull, or intermittent.

Paralysis The inability of a conscious person to move voluntarily is called *paralysis*. It may be caused by a stroke or an injury to the spinal column. If the person has a numbness or t:ngling sensation in the arms or legs, the probability of an injury to the spinal column exists. Ask the conscious victim to grip your hand. Inability to grip signifies partial or complete paralysis.

Vomiting May accompany many conditions, from shock, illness, drowning, and food poisoning, to a simple upset or overloaded stomach. Always ensure an open airway to prevent any aspiration of the vomitus.

Convulsions May occur from an injury or from illness. Ensure an open airway and protect the person from harming himself or herself. Sometimes a soft object such as a rolled up handkerchief or wallet in the corner of the mouth will assist in maintaining an open airway. Do not attempt to restrain a convulsive movement.

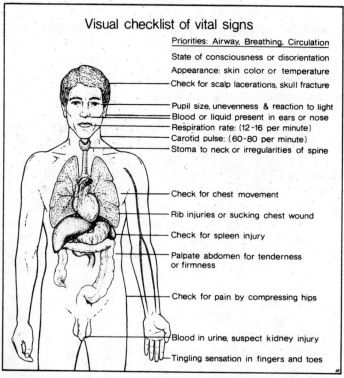

Visual checklist of vital signs

Priorities: Airway, Breathing, Circulation

State of consciousness or disorientation

Appearance: skin color or temperature

Check for scalp lacerations, skull fracture

Pupil size, unevenness & reaction to light

Blood or liquid present in ears or nose

Respiration rate: (12-16 per minute)

Carotid pulse: (60-80 per minute)

Stoma to neck or irregularities of spine

Check for chest movement

Rib injuries or sucking chest wound

Check for spleen injury

Palpate abdomen for tenderness or firmness

Check for pain by compressing hips

Blood in urine, suspect kidney injury

Tingling sensation in fingers and toes

Figure 4 Evaluating the vital signs of an injured person after immediate treatment has been provided. After completing initial examination, continue to observe these signs until medical assistance arrives.

Figure 4, a visual checklist of vital signs, is for evaluating an injured person after immediate treatment has been provided; it encapsulates the material discussed above.

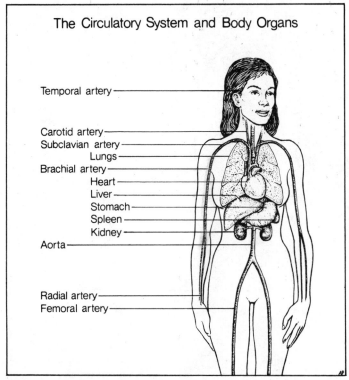

The Circulatory System and Body Organs

Temporal artery

Carotid artery
Subclavian artery
Lungs
Brachial artery
Heart
Liver
Stomach
Spleen
Kidney
Aorta

Radial artery
Femoral artery

Figure 5 Identifying major vessels and organs of the body.

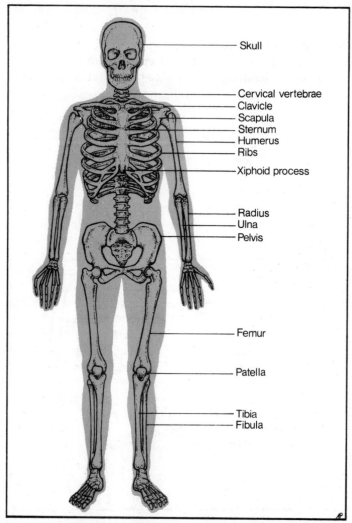

Figure 6 The skeletal system. Identifying principal bones of the body.

When to Call an Ambulance

In most communities an ambulance can be obtained in 10 to 15 minutes or less. If an individual is seriously ill, has heart or breathing problems, has head, neck, or back injuries, or is in severe shock caused by injury, an ambulance should immediately be summoned. If you are in doubt, it is always best to obtain qualified medical rescue assistance.

The Emergency Medical Service system is one of the truly great advances in medical assistance. It extends the hospital emergency department out into the community, and even the wilderness, with trained emergency medical personnel. They are in direct contact with, and/or under the supervision of, the emergency department physician. These specially trained individuals are able to provide basic and advanced life support care, which greatly enhances the victim's chances for survival. Rescues in remote places have been carried out very effectively through search and rescue, helicopter, and other air-sea services. Ideally, in the near future, anywhere within the United States, all emergencies will be able to receive prompt, immediate response by means of the emergency number (911).

Chapter 3
Shock

Shock is caused by a reduction in blood volume in the vital organs and is accompanied by abnormally low blood pressure. Many injuries or conditions may cause a person to go into shock. It may result from severe bleeding, a serious burn, a heart attack, an allergic reaction to a beesting, or heat exhaustion. The excessive loss of body fluids through profuse sweating, diarrhea, or vomiting may also cause shock. Certain signs or symptoms are common to all types of shock (see Figure 1); however, some types of shock have their own specific problems and need special additional treatment.

The degree of shock is usually more severe if a person is bleeding rapidly than if there is a gradual loss of blood. Shock is present in most injuries, but the degree of shock present relates to the overall health, age, and condition of the person involved. In responding to any type of injury it is important to prevent shock from becoming more severe. The first consideration is to treat the injury, then follow other general treatment guidelines for shock. In the recognition of shock it is important to note that all the signs need not be present initially. As

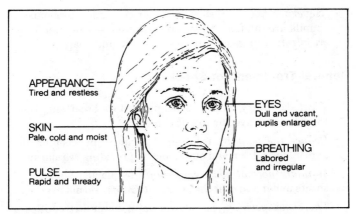

Figure 1 Physical signs and symptoms of shock.

the shock condition persists, more of these signs become evident. If untreated, severe shock may become irreversible and result in death.

As a point of interest, in mild shock, the blood loss from the circulatory system is estimated at 10 to 20 percent; in moderate shock, 20 to 40 percent; and in severe shock, over 40 percent. General guidelines for ascertaining the degree of shock are as follows, although many of these conditions overlap:

Mild Shock Cool skin, paleness, sweating, and signs of thirst; rapid pulse develops and respiratory rate increases.

Moderate Shock Mild conditions become more pronounced; pulse rapid, weak, and thready. Victim tired, restless. Skin becomes cooler, respiration rate increases, breathing may be labored, eyes are dull and vacant, and bluish color of skin develops, especially under fingernails.

Severe Shock Moderate conditions more pronounced; pupils are dilated. There are agitation, stupor, confusion, respiration in gasps, unconsciousness, and death.

General Treatment for Shock

- *Treat the injury,* control bleeding, restore breathing, treat the burn (see specific discussions).
- *Reduce the pain* by treating the injury, by keeping the person lying down and quiet, and by providing reassurance.
- *Maintain normal body temperature* by placing blankets or sheets under and over the person. *Caution:* Do not overheat.
- *The shock position,* i.e., elevation of lower extremities a maximum of 12 inches, will have a temporary effect in increasing amount of blood to vital organs. Do not elevate the legs in the case of head or chest injuries or heart attacks (see Figure 2).
- *Fluids* should never be given if there are suspected head, chest, or abdominal injuries. They are not to be given when emergency medical services are readily available, as in an urban or suburban setting. To relieve the victim's anxieties or a dry, cotton-mouth condition, have the person suck on a damp cloth. In a remote area where medical assistance

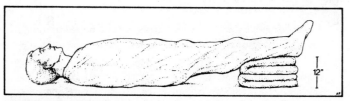

Figure 2 Position for shock if head or chest injuries are not present. Do not elevate if severe leg injuries are present.

is several days away, small amounts of water with a salt solution (1 teaspoon per quart) may be given to the victim. Fluids should be discontinued if the victim becomes nauseated or vomits.

• *Obtain medical assistance.*

Common Types of Shock

Different types of shock require specific treatment in addition to the general recommended treatment. The common types of shock, underlying causes, and specific treatment are:

• *Hemorrhagic* Due to the loss of blood either externally or internally. May also be present in severe contusions and bruises. Follow general shock treatment. This type of shock is also referred to as *hypovolemic.*

• *Anaphylactic* Acute reaction of the body due to a foreign protein entering the system. May be due to injection of drugs, medications, insect stings or bites, etc. Results in paralysis of breathing center if untreated. Treat specific cause, ensure open airway, and administer basic cardiac life support (BCLS) if necessary.

• *Metabolic* Excessive loss of body fluids by vomiting, diarrhea, or dehydration that results in decreased blood volume. Determine cause, increase fluid intake, consider fluid-salt balance in dehydration.

• *Cardiogenic* Due to inadequate functioning of a damaged heart. Cardiopulmonary resuscitation (CPR) may be necessary.

• *Psychogenic* Simple fainting due to temporary reduction of blood supply to the brain. It is not a true state of shock because there is no loss of total blood volume. Determine cause, lay victim in a supine position, and elevate victim's legs to shock position. Cool damp cloth applied to forehead may assist in the victim's response.

Remember, shock due to bleeding, burns, and major injuries is a serious medical emergency. It will be present to some degree after most injuries. The signs may be delayed, *but do not wait until they appear before you provide the recommended treatment.* The severity of shock can be lessened if the victim is given prompt, immediate attention. For this reason the treatment of shock has been given an early priority in this guide.

Chapter 4
Respiratory and Circulatory Emergencies

There are three important considerations when one is dealing with respiratory and circulatory emergencies. They are maintenance of an open airway, adequate breathing, and effective circulation. An obstructed airway may lead to cessation of breathing and heart stoppage. When the heart is not beating, blood cannot circulate to the brain. The cells of the brain will rapidly deteriorate and die if they do not receive oxygen within a 4- to 6-minute period.

Basic Cardiac Life Support

Basic cardiac life support (BCLS) is the lifesaving procedure that consists of the recognition and immediate treatment of a respiratory and circulatory emergency. It should be extended to all individuals who are the victims of heart attacks, drowning, suffocation, anaphylactic shock, drug intoxication, or any instance in which breathing and/or circulation stops. Death often occurs in a heart that is "too good to die" and only needs a second chance to beat! *Training programs in BCLS* (airway management, artificial ventilation or respiration, and cardiopulmonary resuscitation) *are essential in recognizing and providing emergency treatment.* Resuscitation efforts must not await the arrival of trained rescue personnel. If prompt, appropriate application of BCLS is administered, many deaths can be prevented.

In determining a person's need, a specific procedure should be followed. This is referred to as the ABCs of basic cardiac life support: A = airway, B = breathing (respiration), and C = circulation (heart) (see Figure 1).

Unresponsiveness

To test for unresponsiveness in a person, gently shake the victim to awaken him or her unless a neck injury is suspected (Figure 1a). If there is no response, then establish the airway.

Airway

The most important factor for a successful resuscitation is the immediate opening of the airway. This can be accomplished easily by quickly tilting the person's head backward (Figure 1b). This simple maneuver, called the *head tilt–neck lift,* is often all that is required for spontaneous breathing to resume. With the person lying in a supine position, the rescuer places one hand beneath the neck and the other hand on the forehead. The rescuer gently lifts the neck with one hand and tilts the head

Figure 1 Sequence for cardiopulmonary resuscitation (CPR); (a) establish responsiveness; (b) head tilt-neck lift maneuver; (c) observe for signs of breathing; (d) mouth-to-mouth ventilation; (e) feel for carotid pulse; (f) provide external cardiac compression.

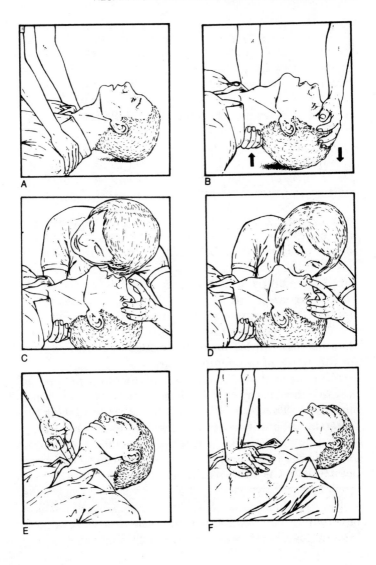

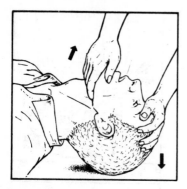

Figure 2 Head tilt–chin lift maneuver.

backward by pressure exerted with the other hand on the forehead. This maneuver extends the neck and lifts the tongue away from the back of the throat. If the victim has dentures, they may be managed with the head tilt–chin lift or taken out. If a neck injury is suspected, *do not overextend the neck* in administering artificial ventilation. To determine whether the victim is breathing, the rescuer looks for the rise and fall of the chest and then listens with an ear to the victim's mouth and nose for indication of breathing (Figure 1c).

The *head tilt–chin lift* is an effective method of opening the airway when the head tilt–neck lift is not successful. This technique is accomplished by placing the fingertips of one hand under the lower jaw (Figure 2), advancing the chin to a forward position. This maneuver supports the lower jaw, although care must be exercised not to compress the soft tissues under the chin, which may obstruct the airway. The other hand presses on the victim's forehead to tilt the head back. The chin should be lifted in such a manner that the teeth are almost brought together; however, the rescuer must avoid closing the mouth altogether. Administer mouth-to-mouth resuscitation if breathing is absent.

Airway Obstruction In a successful resuscitation, the rescuer must always consider the possibility of a foreign body blocking the airway and preventing air from entering the lungs. An obstruction is present if there is a resistance to air flow and a failure of the chest to rise during an attempt to administer artificial ventilation. You will usually know after the first two breaths whether a blockage is present. An important consideration in recognizing an airway obstruction in the conscious person is whether or not the victim can talk. If the victim cannot speak, the eyes bulge, and the person begins to turn a bluish color, an airway obstruction is probably present. The hand clutching the throat is the universal sign of choking (Figure 3).

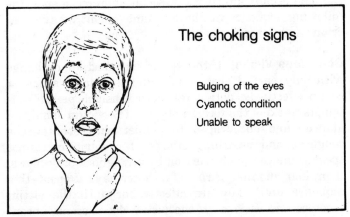

The choking signs

Bulging of the eyes
Cyanotic condition
Unable to speak

Figure 3 The universal distress signal for choking.

Airway Management The methods used in removing an obstruction from the airway of a person are the application of back blows and/or manual abdominal thrusts, and the finger probe. The technique used depends upon whether the victim is conscious or unconscious. If the back blows are unsuccessful, attempt the manual abdominal or chest thrusts. The combination of these two techniques appears to be the most effective method of clearing upper airway obstruction. Repeat the procedure if necessary. *Do not give up.*

If a foreign body is seen in the mouth, attempt to remove it with a finger probe. If it cannot be seen, the combination of back blows and manual thrusts may expel or dislodge it so that it can be removed with the fingers. *Caution:* Use special care in removing a foreign body from the throat of an infant or a small child. An adult's finger may force it deeper into the throat and cause complete airway obstruction.

The American Heart Association recommends the following sequence in airway management for the conscious and unconscious victim.

Conscious Victim If the victim has good air exchange with only partial obstruction, and is able to speak or cough effectively, do not interfere with the person's attempts to expel the foreign object. The victim should be allowed and encouraged to persist with spontaneous coughing and breathing efforts. If the victim cannot speak, remove the obstruction by giving four back blows, then four manual thrusts, if necessary. Repeat this sequence until they are effective or until the victim becomes unconscious. If the victim does become unconscious, repeat these efforts as indicated below.

Unconscious Victim If the victim is unconscious, follow this sequence in determining an airway obstruction. First ventilate. If unsuccessful, reposition the head and try again. If not successful, deliver four back blows, four manual abdominal thrusts, and a finger probe. Next reestablish the airway and attempt to ventilate. If the victim cannot be ventilated, repeat the sequence. When the object has been dislodged provide mouth-to-mouth resuscitation or CPR if necessary. *Note:* As the victim becomes more deprived of oxygen, the muscles tend to relax. Maneuvers that were previously ineffective may become effective. When the muscles relax or a foreign object is partially dislodged, the airway may partially open. Full, slow, and forceful ventilation may keep the victim alive while bypassing the obstruction.

Back-Blow Technique To employ the back-blow technique (Figures 4 and 5), have the person bend head-down, or invert the person over a chair, or roll him or her into

Figure 4 Back-blow technique, bent-down position.

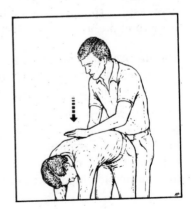

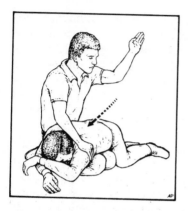

Figure 5 Back-blow technique, supine position.

your lap. Place one hand on the breastbone (sternum) and with the other hand deliver four firm blows between the shoulder blades in rapid succession. Each back blow should be administered with the intention of relieving the obstruction. Return the person back to the original position and sweep the obstruction out of the mouth with your fingers. If not successful, repeat the procedure. For best results, the head should be lower then the rest of the body to make use of the effects of gravity.

Manual Abdominal Thrusts   Deliver manual thrusts to the upper abdomen at a 45° angle in either a standing, sitting, or supine position (lying on the back).

Standing or Sitting Position   Stand behind the person and wrap your arms around the victim's waist (Figure 6). Be sure your chest is firmly against the person's back with your head slightly to the side. Place the fist with the thumb side against the abdomen, slightly above the

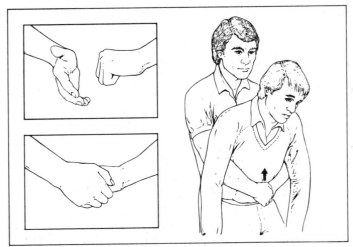

Figure 6 Manual abdominal thrusts, standing position.

navel (under the diaphragm) and below the rib cage and tip of the sternum. Grasp the fist with the other hand and press firmly into the person's abdomen with quick upward thrusts four times. Repeat this procedure if necessary. Do not apply any pressure to the rib cage.

Supine Position   With the person lying on the back, kneel facing the victim astride one thigh or the hips (Figure 7). You may also align your knees to either side of the victim near the hips. Place one hand on top of the other hand with the heel of the bottom hand on the abdomen, slightly above the navel and below the rib cage. Press into the abdomen with quick upward thrusts four times. Repeat this procedure if necessary.

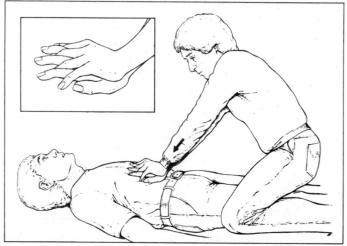

Figure 7 Manual abdominal thrusts, supine position.

Chest Thrusts The chest thrust is the preferred method of relieving a foreign obstruction if there is marked obesity or advanced pregnancy (Figure 8). To apply the chest thrust, stand behind the victim with your arms directly under the victim's armpits, encircling the chest. Place the thumb side of the fist at midsternum (avoiding the margins of the rib cage and the xiphoid process), grasp that fist with the other hand, and exert four backward thrusts. If possible the victim should be leaning forward to make the most effective use of gravity. If the victim is in a supine position, this maneuver is similar to that used during external chest compression.

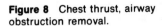

Figure 8 Chest thrust, airway obstruction removal.

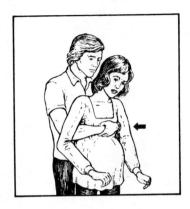

Finger Probe   Open the victim's mouth by grasping both the tongue and lower jaw between your thumb and fingers and lift. This action, called the *tongue-jaw lift,* draws the tongue away from the back of the throat and away from a foreign object. This technique may partially relieve the obstruction. Next, insert the index finger down along the inside of the cheeks and deeply into the throat to the base of the tongue. Then use a hooking motion to dislodge the foreign object and maneuver it into the mouth for removal. *Be careful not to force the object deeper into the airway.* If the foreign object comes within reach, grasp and remove it. (See Figure 9.)

Breathing

If the victim does not promptly resume adequate, spontaneous breathing after the airway is opened, artificial ventilation (rescue breathing) must be initiated. Mouth-

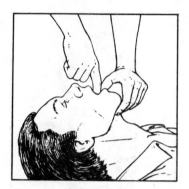

Figure 9 Finger probe for foreign object.

to-mouth or mouth-to-nose breathing are the two best types of artificial ventilation.

    Mouth-to-Mouth Ventilation In performing *mouth-to-mouth ventilation,* use the head tilt technique of placing one hand under the person's head. With the other hand, pinch the nostrils together with the thumb and index finger. The heel of this hand exerts pressure on the forehead to ensure an adequate airway. Take a deep breath, then open your mouth and place it firmly on the victim's mouth. Administer four quick, full breaths without waiting for the person's lungs to deflate between breaths. After delivering these breaths, check the carotid pulse. If a pulse is present, indicating a heartbeat, one deep breath should be given every 5 seconds, or 12 breaths per minute. Remove your mouth between breaths so the person can exhale. Adequate breathing is monitored on every breath by watching for the rise and fall of the chest, feeling in your own airway the resistance of the person's lungs as they expand, and hearing and feeling the air escape during exhalation.

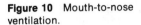

Figure 10 Mouth-to-nose ventilation.

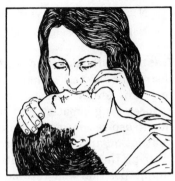

Mouth-to-Nose Ventilation Use *mouth-to-nose ventilation* if the person has facial injuries or has taken a corrosive poison or if a good seal cannot be formed (Figure 10). In the mouth-to-nose method, tilt the head back with one hand on the forehead and with the other hand lift the jaw. Blow into the person's nose, using your cheek to close off the mouth, or hold the chin closed with the hand that is not on the victim's forehead. It may be necessary to open the person's mouth to allow air to escape between breaths.

Mouth-to-Stoma Ventilation This type of artificial ventilation is used for a person who had a laryngectomy (a neck breather) and has an open stoma (permanent hole) in the neck. Do not tilt the head; ventilate directly into the tube or stoma of the neck.

The most common faults in administering artificial respiration are these:

- Inadequate head tilt
- Not properly pinching the nose

- Not forming a good seal around the mouth
- Not administering enough air during ventilation

Gastric Distension and Vomiting It is not unusual for distension of the stomach to occur in small children or even adults. Excessive distension of the stomach reduces lung capacity and induces vomiting and subsequent aspiration of the fluids. If vomiting occurs, stop ventilation and turn the person's entire body to the side, clearing the mouth of vomitus. Return the victim to the supine position and resume CPR. *Note:* If the stomach becomes distended during rescue breathing, avoid excessive airway pressure by repositioning the airway and carefully observing the rise and fall of the chest. Continue the rescue breathing without attempting to relieve the stomach contents. Compression on the upper abdomen may cause the victim to regurgitate and aspirate some of the stomach contents into the lungs. Relief of gastric distension should be attempted only if the abdomen is so tense that ventilation is ineffective. This is the case whether the victim is an adult, a child, or an infant. If it is necessary to relieve gastric distension, turn the entire body to the side prior to applying pressure to the upper abdomen. After compressing the stomach, wipe all vomitus out of the mouth and return the victim to his or her back to resume CPR.

Circulation

The absence of the carotid pulse in the neck indicates a lack of blood flow and no heartbeat. Thus, we enter into the third consideration in dealing with respiratory and circulatory emergencies—cardiopulmonary resuscitation, or CPR.[1]

CPR   In the rescue, the rescuer compresses on the victim's chest, forcing blood out of the heart to the brain and other vital organs. This is called *external cardiac compression* (ECC) and must be accompanied by artificial ventilation. CPR consists of opening and maintaining an airway, providing artificial ventilation by rescue breathing, and creating artificial circulation by external cardiac compression. AR + ECC = CPR.

Before performing CPR, the rescuer must be able to recognize the need, understand the potential risks during performance, and have practiced the resuscitative skills. In determining the need, the rescue person should always follow the set procedure of gently shaking the victim[2] and/or shouting to determine consciousness, opening the airway, giving four quick breaths, and checking the carotid pulse for a heart beat (see the accompanying Checklist). Further assessments may include checking for lack of movement in the victim, for unusual color of the skin (paleness or bluish tint, especially under the fingernails), and the size of the pupils.

Hazards during CPR   Potential risks are involved during the performance of CPR (Figure 11). While these complications may occur even with the best of performances,

---

[1] Procedures on CPR adapted from *A Manual for Instructors of Basic Life Support,* American Heart Association, Dallas, Tex., 1977, from the 1980 updated edition, and from "Standards and Guidelines for Cardiopulmonary Resuscitation (CPR) and Emergency Cardiac Care (ECC)," *Journal of the American Medical Association,* vol. 244, no. 5, 1980.

[2] Do not shake if neck injury is suspected.

careful attention to details of technique during performance will minimize the problems. Listed are potential hazards associated with inadequate performance:

- Pressure over the xiphoid process (tip of sternum) may lacerate the liver.
- Pressure with the fingers on the rib cage may cause rib fractures and punctured lung.
- Pressure too high on the sternum may cause fracture of the sternum.
- Pressure at an angle other than 90° may fracture ribs or sternum or may lacerate the heart.
- Insufficient pressure is ineffective in providing enough cardiac output.
- Jerky movements increase the risk of fractures of the rib or sternum and do not enhance blood flow or blood pressure.
- Pressure to sternum and abdomen or stomach at the same time may lead to the rupture of the liver and/or the stomach. It may also lead to regurgitation and aspiration of stomach contents.

Performance of CPR In the performance of CPR, the victim must be on a firm surface. Kneel close to the side of the victim, placing one hand over the other, and on the lower half of the sternum. Your hand should be on the sternum and approximately 2 inches above the xiphoid process (see Figure 12). Pressure on the sternum compresses the heart against the spinal column, forcing the blood out of the heart and providing circulation. The flow of blood resulting from this compression is approximately one-fourth to one-third of the normal cardiac output,

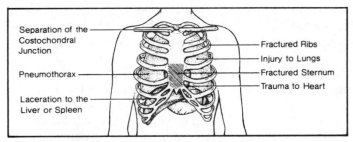

Figure 11 Potential risks in performing CPR.

enough to sustain life. The depth of the compression is $1\frac{1}{2}$ to 2 inches in adults, and $\frac{3}{4}$ to $1\frac{1}{2}$ inches in children. The compressions must be regular, smooth, and uninterrupted. Relaxation must immediately follow compression and be of equal duration (50 percent of the cycle should be compression and 50 percent should be relaxation). For the proper hand position, the heel of the hand must

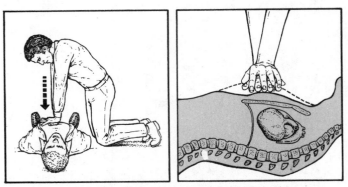

Figure 12 Proper position for external cardiac compression.

remain in contact with the sternum; however, all pressure is released on the upstroke to allow maximum refilling of the heart. In the single-person rescue, a 15:2 ratio is performed (15 compressions in 11 to 12 seconds and then 2 quick ventilations in 3 to 4 seconds). The rate for the single-rescue person is 80 per minute, to allow time for the ventilation (Figure 13). In the two-person rescue the ratio is 5:1 at a rate of 60 per minute (five compressions to one ventilation). The advantage of the two-person rescue is that blood flow can remain constant while the ventilations are delivered. The rescuers work on opposite sides and can exchange positions without disturbing the rhythm of the performance, sustaining their rescue operation for a longer time (Figure 14). The ventilator must be ready to quickly interpose the single breath as

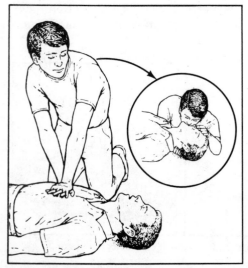

Figure 13 Single-person rescue CPR.

the compressor releases the pressure from the fifth compression. This permits the maximum ventilation of air into the lungs. CPR should not be stopped for over 5 seconds and should be continued until the victim is transferred to the care of trained medical personnel. The carotid pulse should be checked for 5 seconds after the first minute of CPR and every few minutes thereafter to review the effectiveness of CPR and the status of the person. An additional assessment of the victim's pulse should be made when a second rescuer arrives at the scene. The reaction of the pupils should also be periodically examined, as they are the best indicator of oxygenated blood being delivered to the victim's brain. Other signs of effective resuscitation include the rising and falling of the person's chest, improvement of skin color, and any purposeful movement.

Once breathing has been restored in any resuscitation effort, place the victim in a comfortable position, usually on the side or with the head and shoulders slightly elevated. Treat for shock during and after any respiratory emergency and refer to a physician.

CPR CHECKLIST

Single-Person Rescue	Two-Person Rescue
Determine consciousness	Determine consciousness
Extend airway	Extend airway
Four quick ventilations	Four quick ventilations
Check carotid pulse	Check carotid pulse
Apply 15 compressions (11–12 per second)	Apply 5 compressions (1 per second)
2 quick ventilations	1 quick ventilation (on fifth upstroke)
Repeat cycle at 15:2 ratio	Repeat cycle at 5:1 ratio

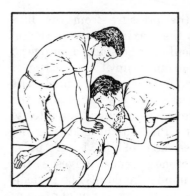

Figure 14 Two-person rescue CPR. *(Note:* During the exchange of positions the rescuers pause for 5 seconds after the 5:1 sequence, and the compressor rechecks the pulse. The ventilator moves into position to resume the compressions if necessary and to continue CPR.)

The Cough as a CPR Technique[3] The cough is an effective method of providing CPR to the conscious person experiencing a heart attack. A forceful and repeated cough every 1 to 3 seconds ensures breathing, can return the pulse, and can maintain normal blood pressure. The cough is produced by a strong contraction of the diaphragm and intercostal muscles while the glottis is closed. This procedure enhances thoracic pressure similar to external cardiac compression. The cough is easy to perform in any position and does not require a firm surface. Rhythmic coughing is a simple procedure that may "buy time" for the conscious person having a heart attack until medical assistance can be obtained.

[3] Adapted from Paul E. Fenster, M.D., and Gordon A. Ewy, M.D., "Cardiopulmonary Resuscitation: Recent Insights and New Developments," *Practical Cardiology,* vol. 6, no. 5, 1980.

Resuscitation, Airway Management, and CPR for Infants and Children

Resuscitation Determine whether an infant or child is unconscious by gently tapping or shaking. The conscious infant or child will begin to move or cry. If the child is not unconscious but gasping to breathe, it is necessary to open the airway and coordinate your breathing with the child's. The opening of the airway and administering of artificial ventilation are essentially the same for infants and children as for adults (Figure 15). Care must be taken with infants not to overextend the neck and thereby close off the airway. Ventilation is performed by covering both the mouth and the nose at the same time with your mouth. Smaller amounts of air are given, only small puffs, with one breath every 3 seconds, a rate of 20 per minute. In children the rate of respiration is approximately 16 per minute.

Checking the Pulse The child's pulse can be felt over the carotid artery, just as in the adult. The infant's pulse

Figure 15 Artificial ventilation, infant.

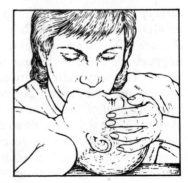

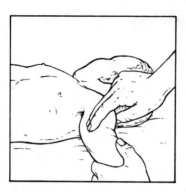

Figure 16 Checking brachial pulse, infant.

can be felt on the brachial artery as the carotid is difficult to locate. This pulse is located on the inside of the upper arm midway between the shoulder and elbow (Figure 16). *Note:* The carotid pulse is difficult to locate in the infant due to the short and sometimes fat neck. The apical pulse is not considered to be a reliable pulse as it represents precordial activity and an impulse rather than a pulse.

Airway Management The same technique for removing an airway obstruction with back blows applies to infants (Figure 17). Invert the infant and hold the head down. Support the head with your hand around the jaws and chest. You may gain additional support by resting your forearm on your thigh. Deliver four back blows rapidly with the heel of the hand between the infant's shoulder blades. After the back blows are delivered, the infant is turned and placed on the rescuer's thigh and given four chest thrusts in rapid succession. The chest thrusts are performed in the same manner as that in which external

Figure 17 Back blows, infant (airway obstruction).

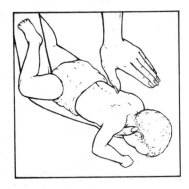

chest compressions are applied to the infant. (Abdominal thrusts are not recommended for infants and children because of the potential danger of injury to the abdominal organs, especially the liver.) If the victim is a child, turn him or her over your thigh (with the head lower than the trunk) and deliver four back blows with somewhat greater force than that used for the infant. Next, roll the child over on the floor (supporting the head) and give four chest thrusts in the same manner as that in which external chest compression is performed on the adult. After completing the chest thrusts, remove the foreign object from the infant or child by sweeping the fingers through the mouth. Be careful not to force the object deeper into the throat. *Note:* The infant who has only a *partial* airway obstruction and who is moving some air should not be turned upside down for removal of a foreign object. Turning the infant upside down may bring about a complete airway obstruction, causing the foreign object to become impacted against the undersurface of the vocal cords.

CPR for Infants and Children   With a few exceptions, external cardiac compression is the same for children as for adults. For small children, the heel of one hand is used during the compression. Compress the sternum $\frac{3}{4}$ to $1\frac{1}{2}$ inches. With infants, only the tips of the index and middle fingers are used (Figure 18). Compression of $\frac{1}{2}$ to $\frac{3}{4}$ inches at midsternum should be exerted at the rate of 100 compressions per minute. With the infant, the rescuer uses a 5:1 ratio and interposes the one small breath between each five compressions.

Note: An infant is generally defined as anyone under 1 year of age. A child is defined as anyone between 1 and 8 years of age. For a victim above 8 years of age, the same techniques usually apply that are appropriate for adults.

Other Considerations for CPR

- If a neck injury is suspected due to the nature of the accident, special caution must be given in administering artificial ventilation.

- The person lying in the prone position should be turned

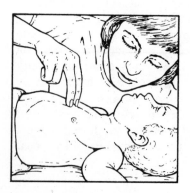

Figure 18   CPR, Infant.

carefully to the supine position. Special care must be used during this turn to prevent injury to the neck. CPR can only be performed with the victim in the supine position.

- Medical help must be summoned immediately (emergency medical services, fire department, etc.). Continue CPR until rescue personnel arrive.

- If the victim vomits, stop your efforts, turn the head and the entire body on to the side, and clear out the throat.

- Sustain your efforts longer with children, under cold weather conditions, and with drowning victims (successful rescues have been reported from 30 minutes up to several hours depending on climatic conditions and the overall health of the person).

- The sooner CPR is initiated, the greater are the chances of survival and the less the chance of brain damage.

- Many rescue attempts will be unsuccessful, but the alternative to not performing CPR, if needed, is certain death.

- Remember, CPR is not begun until it is ascertained that the victim does not show evidence of breathing or have a pulse.

The procedures indicated for CPR will serve as a reference for its proper application. They should not be substituted for a training program, which is essential in learning this lifesaving technique. Enroll in a course in CPR from the local American Heart Association or American Red Cross.

Drowning

Drowning is one of the leading causes of accidental death in the United States. Most of these deaths could be prevented if individuals would develop a sound approach to, and a healthy respect for, the water. Listed are some "commonsense" safety precautions that should be followed:

- Learn to swim, tread water, and relax around the water.
- Know your abilities and limitations. *Do not* swim alone.
- Orient and care for children around the water.
- Adjust slowly to cool or cold water; do not swim if overly tired.
- Follow the safety rules of the area, beach, or pool.
- Do not swim or dive in unknown waters. Swim only in supervised areas.
- Do not swim in areas where riptides or strong undercurrents are present.
- Follow the U.S. Coast Guard rules on boating safety. (These may be obtained from U.S. Coast Guard District Office or Auxiliary).
- Do not get careless in boats by standing up, or while changing positions or untangling fishing lines.[4]
- If a boat overturns, stay with the boat.
- If a storm is brewing, seek the closest shore.
- Do not cross swollen streams or river beds.
- Do not camp in areas where flashflooding may occur.
- When rescuing a person, use good judgment. Extend a flotation device, rope, towel, fishing pole, or similar object, especially if you are not trained in lifesaving techniques.
- If a person has possible neck injuries, use a backboard or

[4] A common cause of men falling overboard is standing up to urinate. It is recommended that you carry an extra cup or get to shore for this duty.

surfboard for support prior to removing that person from the water.

- Never swim underwater for long distances, even if you are an expert swimmer. When swimming underwater for long distances, a person may black out and drown without any warning.

Acute asphyxia (suffocation) occurs in all drowning or near-drowning people. The airway to the lungs becomes clogged with water and death may result from lack of oxygen. The drowning person will often have a substantial amount of water in the stomach, and vomiting is likely to occur during resuscitation. If vomiting occurs, stop resuscitation. Turn the victim onto the side and clear out the mouth. Return the victim to the supine position and resume artificial respiration.

Treatment Initially give the person four quick breaths. Do not wait until you reach the shore. As you are bringing the person to the shore, continue artificial respiration. If there is no pulse present, give CPR. *Note:* CPR cannot be given in the water, as a firm surface is necessary to perform it. If the victim recovers, turn him or her onto the side, treat for shock, and seek medical assistance.

Chapter 5
Wounds and Related Injuries

A victim with severe bleeding is considered a critical case in emergency medical care. The bleeding may be external or internal. The sooner the bleeding is controlled, the less urgent the problem. External bleeding can usually be controlled. Most internal bleeding, however, is difficult to control, and is a serious medical emergency.

External Bleeding

The general objectives in the management of all serious wounds are to *control the bleeding, prevent infection,* and *treat for shock.* The most effective method of controlling external bleeding is to apply direct pressure at the site of the bleeding or hemorrhaging (*bleeding* and *hemorrhaging* are synonymous). The body of the average adult contains approximately 6 liters of blood (1 liter = 1.0567 quarts). The loss of a single quart can result in serious shock. Continued loss can cause death. For example, if bleeding from a major artery is not controlled, a person may bleed to death in less than 3 minutes. The most

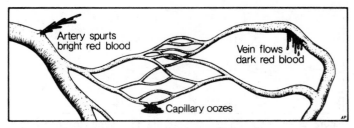

Figure 1 Blood flow sequence: artery-capillary-vein.

important consideration in any serious bleeding, regardless of the type of vessel, is to control it as soon as possible. In most severe external wounds it is likely that an artery, veins, and capillaries all have been injured (see Figure 1). The bleeding from an artery will *spurt* bright red, freshly oxygenated blood. The bleeding from a vein is slower and the blood is of a darker color. It is serious but usually easier to control. The bleeding from capillaries *oozes* and is less profuse and less serious. Generally speaking, the bleeding of a completely severed artery is easier to control than one that is only partly severed. In a completely severed artery, the elasticity of the walls of the vessel will cause the ends to close off, decreasing the flow of the blood from the opening. With bleeding from a vessel that is only partly severed this does not occur. The elasticity of the severed vessel parts tends to cause them to pull away from each other, increasing the opening of the vessel and the flow of blood.

The sequence in controlling severe bleeding of external wounds is: *pressure bandage, pressure points, constricting band,* and *tourniquet.*

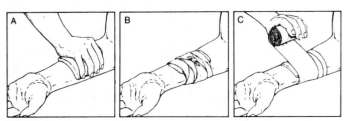

Figure 2 (a) Applying direct pressure to wound. (b) Applying a pressure bandage to wound. (c) The elastic bandage as a pressure bandage.

Pressure Bandage A pressure bandage is the most effective method of controlling any external bleeding. Apply a firm, steady pressure directly over the wound with the cleanest possible bandage (see Figure 2a and b). Use a dry, sterile dressing (DSD) if possible. Maintain this pressure until the bleeding slows or stops. A slight elevation of the injured part may aid in the control of the bleeding. Secure the bandage with a cravat or an elastic bandage. The knot of the cravat should be secured directly over the wound. This will provide additional pressure to the wound. This technique should be applied to all bleeding wounds except injuries to the eye, or in the case of an object embedded or impaled in the injury. In applying a pressure bandage with the elastic bandage, do not secure it too tightly as it may cut off the circulation of the area below the wound (see Figure 2c). The initial wraps should be snug but not tight, in case a part of the bandage needs to be loosened and reapplied. *The bandage is too tight if the pulse cannot be felt below the injury.* Sometimes, however, a weak pulse cannot be felt in any case. An overly tight bandage may also result in bluish coloration or throbbing of the affected part.

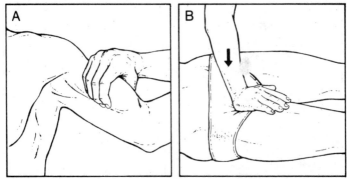

Figure 3 The major pressure points to assist in controlling arterial bleeding are (a) the brachial artery, and (b) the femoral artery.

Pressure Points A pressure point is any point where an artery can be felt or where it passes directly over a bone. The artery can be compressed to help control bleeding distal to (beyond) that point. The combined use of the pressure point with a direct pressure bandage to the wound will normally control all external bleeding. Use pressure points to help control serious bleeding. Pressure should be applied to the brachial artery (upper arm, see Figure 3a) and to the femoral artery (upper leg, see Figure 3b). Additional pressure points may be used on the temporal and the subclavian vessels (see Figure 4a and b).

Constricting Band A constricting band may be used to aid in the control of bleeding from an arm or leg while the pressure bandage is applied. Place a cravat bandage or similar object firmly around the extremity. It should be applied several inches above the wound with the knot

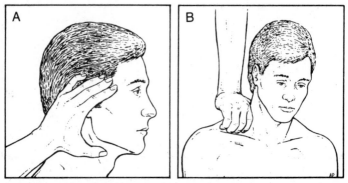

Figure 4 Additional pressure points include (a) the temporal artery and (b) the subclavian artery.

or tie over the supplying artery (see Figure 5a). To determine appropriate tightness, check to ensure that you can insert your finger under the band. After the pressure bandage has been applied, the constricting band should be removed. The constricting band is also used for snakebite injuries.

Tourniquet The application of a tourniquet (TQ) is seldom necessary. It should not be used unless the arm or leg has been mangled so badly that the bleeding cannot be controlled by any other method. Severed parts can be reattached through microscopic surgery, but the application of a tourniquet makes this procedure virtually impossible because of the destruction of the body tissue. If the tourniquet is applied, it should be placed 2 to 3 inches above the wound with the knot over the supplying artery. Tighten gently, just until the bleeding stops (see

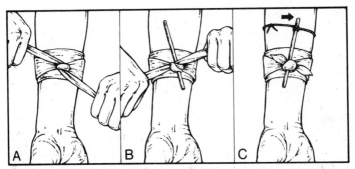

Figure 5 (*a*) The application of the constricting band. (*b*) By continuing to tighten the constricting band it becomes a tourniquet. (*c*) Securing the tourniquet.

Figure 5*b* and *c*). Note the time the TQ was applied. *Do not* remove without medical advice.

Note: Any completely severed part should be placed in a cold, wet cloth or a plastic container with cold water. This is a necessary procedure to preserve the severed part and make a successful replant possible.

Treatment of Severe Wounds

All open wounds are subject to infection. Special precautions must be taken to prevent contamination. The general procedures for severe-wound management are:

- Place the cleanest possible material over the wound (dry, sterile dressing) and secure with a pressure bandage.
- Immobilize the area or the part. Keep the person still and lying down.

- Do not cleanse the wound if medical care is readily available.
- Elevate the part to heart level, unless other injuries preclude this.
- Treat for shock.
- Arrange transportation to the hospital.

Prevention of Infection   Cleanliness is the most important safeguard against infection. All minor wounds should be cleansed thoroughly after the bleeding has been controlled. Essential procedures for cleansing wounds are:

- Wash the wound thoroughly with warm water and a mild soap. Wash away from the wound to prevent further contamination.
- Small objects may be removed by tweezers. Any deeply embedded objects should be removed by a physician.
- Rinse the wound thoroughly with cool water.
- Dry the area by patting with a DSD or clean cloth.
- Application of a mild antiseptic solution is permissible. Avoid first-aid creams as they tend to keep the wound moist.
- Place a DSD over the wound, then bandage it. Allow the wound to breathe by not completely enclosing it. This will allow it to scab over (see Figure 6).
- If there is a danger of the wound becoming dirty, then it should be completely closed.
- Be sure to consult with your physician about a tetanus booster, especially if the injury occurs around animals.

The danger of infection is always present in all wounds. This is especially the case in wounds that do not bleed

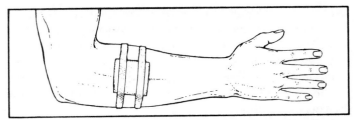

Figure 6 Applying a dry, sterile dressing and securing with adhesive tape.

freely or that contain embedded objects such as dirt, cinder, glass, or splinters.

Signs Tenderness, throbbing pain, swelling, and redness of the affected part. Evidence of pus draining from the wound. Fever, swollen lymph glands, and red streaks leading from the wound indicate that an infection is present (see "Cellulitis," Chapter 13).

Treatment Obtain prompt medical care for all infected wounds. An antibiotic may be necessary to control infection. If medical assistance is not readily available, apply very warm soaks or moist, hot towels frequently to the area. Elevate the body part and keep the person quiet.

Classification of Wounds: Open Wounds

In an open wound there is always a break in the skin and tissue damage. Some wounds are more serious than others and require specific treatment. Open wounds are classified as *abrasions, incisions, lacerations, punctures,* and *avulsions.*

Abrasion An abrasion occurs when the outer layers of the skin are scraped against hard surfaces. Examples of abrasions are skinned knees and elbows and floor burns. Bleeding is usually limited to oozing of blood from the small capillaries. The greatest danger is contamination of the wound by dirt and bacteria ground into the tissue.

Treatment Initially control the bleeding with a light pressure bandage. Wash the wound thoroughly with warm water and a mild soap. Wash away from the wound, removing all foreign objects. Hydrogen peroxide is a good cleansing agent. Apply a mild antiseptic to the wound and allow to dry. Cover the wound with a DSD, allowing the wound to breathe and scab over. Refer to a physician if foreign objects are embedded in the wound.

Incision An incision is a single, clean cut. The cut may occur from a sharp object, such as a knife or broken glass, and bleeds freely. The cut, if serious, may damage muscle, tendon, and other tissue.

Treatment Control the bleeding with a pressure bandage. Any severe cut should be seen by a physician for possible suturing. If you can remove the object without further injury, do so. For minor cuts, after bleeding has been controlled, cleanse the wound thoroughly with soap and water. Apply a butterfly bandage and a DSD.

Laceration A laceration or lacerated wound is usually a jagged or irregular injury. It is often due to extreme force, and bleeding may be severe. It may be contaminated by foreign objects. Lacerations may occur from blunt objects, from an automobile, or in virtually any accident situation.

Treatment   Initially control the bleeding with a pressure bandage. In minor lacerations, cleanse the wound thoroughly with soap and water. Use the butterfly bandage and apply a DSD. On any wound that may leave a scar, refer to a physician for possible suturing.

Puncture   A puncture wound is caused by a sharp object which penetrates the body tissue. Injuries of this type do not bleed freely, and infection is a concern. Puncture situations include stepping on a nail, animal bites, and slivers.

Treatment   Initially control any minor bleeding with a DSD. If the object is not embedded, soak the affected part in very warm water 15 to 20 minutes, three to four times daily. Apply a DSD over the wound, allowing the wound to breathe. Be sure the victim's tetanus shot is up to date.

Avulsion   An avulsion is caused by a forceful tearing or separation of tissue from the body. It is often accompanied by severe bleeding. Avulsions may be caused by explosions, automobile accidents, and animal bites. They are usually very serious injuries.

Treatment   Control the bleeding with a direct-pressure bandage. If any part of the body has been torn off, place it in a clean, damp, cool cloth and take it with you to the hospital.

Internal Bleeding

Internal bleeding as evidenced by shock requires immediate medical attention. The bleeding may occur in the chest, the abdominal cavity, or the pelvic area. It may be caused by a severed artery or an injury to a vital organ such as the liver, spleen, or kidney. Internal bleeding of this nature often results from crush injuries or automobile accidents.

Signs Moderate to severe shock conditions may be present, such as irregular breathing and thready pulse rate, restlessness, faintness, cold clammy skin, dilated pupils, dizziness, and thirst. The following signs may suggest an injury to a specific vital organ:

- *Lungs* Coughing up of bright red, frothy blood
- *Stomach or throat* Vomiting bright red blood
- *Spleen* Firmness of the muscles and a dull pain on the left side toward the back (below rib cage)
- *Kidneys* Blood in the urine
- *Intestines* Blood in the stools

Treatment Seek immediate medical attention. Treat for shock.

Classification of Wounds: Closed Wounds

A closed wound is one in which the blood vessels have been ruptured, usually in the muscle or a joint area. There is a leakage of blood and other fluid into the tissue and it has the appearance of being "black-and-blue." The bleeding is usually limited and the skin unbroken. Bruises, strains, and sprains are examples of closed wounds.

Bruises   A bruise (*contusion*) is usually caused by a fall or a blow to the body. The capillaries are ruptured and the blood oozes into the tissue. Initially the bruise is red and swollen to some degree, depending upon severity.

Signs   Swelling, tenderness, pain, and a black-and-blue appearance. In severe bruises, shock may be present.

Treatment   Apply a cold compress or ice bag to the area for 20 to 25 minutes three or four times daily. After removing the cold compress, apply a pressure bandage and elevate the part if possible. Prescribe rest and limit activity. After 48 hours or so, heat or warm soaks may be applied. Severe bruises should be seen by a physician.

Bleeding from the Head or Scalp

Any injury to the scalp usually bleeds freely. There are many blood vessels located in the scalp.

Treatment   The bleeding of any scalp wound can usually be controlled with a direct-pressure bandage. Special care, however, must be provided if there are any bony fragments present. Apply the pressure dressing and secure with a roller bandage to control the bleeding. Keep the person still and obtain medical assistance.

Bleeding from the Neck

Any bleeding wound from the neck is a serious medical emergency. Cover the wound with a sterile bandage of several thicknesses. Maintain firm pressure on the wound to control bleeding. *Do not* encircle the neck with the bandage. Provide special care in maintaining an open airway for breathing and removing any blood that may collect in the throat. Do not overlook the possibility of a fractured neck. Obtain medical assistance.

Bleeding from the Chest

Puncture wounds of the chest may cause what is known as a *sucking chest wound* (see Figure 7). If an object penetrates deep into the lungs, it will have entered the pleural cavity. It may cause a collapse of the lung. *Caution:* Do not remove any penetrating object, as it may increase the bleeding and loss of air from the lung.

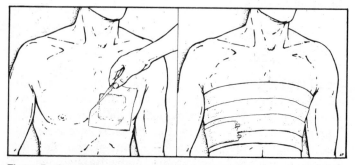

Figure 7 A sucking chest wound. Apply gauze dressing, plastic wrap, and roller bandage.

Signs Sucking sound upon inhalation. Bleeding is usually present. The person is likely to cough up frothy, bright blood.

Treatment Immediately seal off the wound with an airtight dressing. Use a petroleum jelly gauze dressing, plastic covering, or thin plastic film (e.g., Saran Wrap) and roller bandage over the dressing. The dressing must be large enough so that it will not be sucked into the opening. Secure a large bandage, cravat, or pressure bandage over the injury. Lay the person on the injured side and arrange for transportation to a hospital. *Note:* Encourage the victim to cough up any blood or secretions from the air passages.

Stove-In Chest

In automobile accidents, a person who smashes into the steering wheel may sustain a crushing injury to the chest. (Also suspect a spinal injury.) The victim may experience difficulty in breathing because of fractured ribs or a punctured lung. Multiple rib fractures may cause a collapse of part of the chest. This is referred to as a *flail* or *stove-in chest*. With the flail chest the sternum is "floating" and often the chest needs to be held down to assist breathing.

Treatment Place the person in a position where he or she can breathe easily (semirecumbent or on the injured side). Any open wound should be bandaged. Allow the person to spit out any blood coughed up from the lungs. Do not splint the rib cage if medical help is available.

Treat for shock and obtain medical assistance. *Note:* If the pain is severe enough to cause the victim problems in breathing, place your hand on the person's chest with 5 to 10 pounds of pressure. This will enable the victim to breathe more easily. It may be necessary to turn the person onto the injured side to prevent the ribs from moving in and out during respiration.

Bleeding from the Abdomen

In serious abdominal wounds the intestines or other vital organs may be exposed. This may result from a violent automobile accident or a gunshot wound. This is a serious medical emergency. Obtain an ambulance immediately.

Signs Exposed intestines and other organs. Severe bleeding may be present.

Treatment Try to control the bleeding by applying light pressure with several thicknesses of a sterile gauze. Cover the protruding intestines with a damp cloth. Treat for shock and obtain medical assistance. *Note:* All gunshot wounds must be reported to the police.

Nosebleed

A nosebleed is common and may be caused by a blow to the nasal area or by excessive blowing of the nose.

Signs Bleeding from the nose.

Treatment Place the person in a sitting position, leaning slightly forward with the head bowed. Pinch or squeeze the nostrils together, applying firm pressure. Apply a cold compress (ice bag) across the bridge of the nose for 5 to 6 minutes. It will usually control the bleeding. If bleeding does not stop after 15 to 30 minutes, insert a small wad of sterile gauze up the nostril and repeat the cold applications with pressure to the nose. Leave the gauze in the nose for several hours if necessary. *Do not blow the nose.* Encourage the person to spit out any blood that may drain back into the throat.

Other Injuries

Not all injuries can be neatly categorized. Such is the case with the following injuries, which range from head to toe and from minor to serious.

Injuries to the Eyes Foreign bodies such as dust or small dirt particles lodged in the eyes are usually easy to remove. They are commonly found under the upper lid and are extremely irritating. Do not rub the eye as that may cause further injury. To determine the location of a foreign object in the eye, lift the upper lid by grasping the eyelash and pulling outward. If this relieves the pain, the object is probably sticking to the inside of the eyelid.

Object on the Inside of the Eyelid To remove the object, turn the upper lid inside out by grasping the lashes with the eye looking down (see Figure 8). Press down on

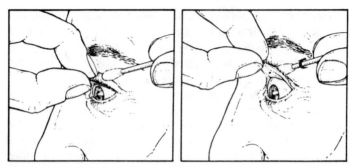

Figure 8 Foreign object in the eye. Invert eyelid with cotton-tipped applicator.

the middle of the lid with a cotton swab and evert the lid over the cotton swab. The object may be on the inside of the eyelid. Gently remove the object with a clean, moist, sterile applicator, or the corner of a moist handkerchief. *Caution:* Do not rub the eye.

Object on the Eyeball If the object can be seen on the clear surface of the eye, have the victim attempt to dislodge it by blinking the eye or by using a gentle stream of water to rinse it off (use an eyedropper if available).

Scratched Eyeball If the eyeball has been scratched, it will usually be irritated for several days. Apply a soft, wet tissue or cloth and cover with a DSD. Refer the victim to a physician.

Embedded Object If a foreign body is embedded in the eye, *do not disturb the object*. It should be removed only by a physician, preferably an ophthalmologist. Cover the eye socket with a small "gauze doughnut" to prevent the object from being pressed into the eye. Cover both eyes, for they move together, and this will prevent any motion of the injured eye (see Figure 9). Covering both eyes is sometimes frightening to the victim. Explain the reason for covering the eyes and give reassurance. Seek immediate medical attention.

Laceration of the Eyelids Any cuts around the eye must be handled with extreme care. A small pressure bandage will normally control any bleeding. Examine the injury carefully prior to applying the pressure bandage to the eye. Be sure there are no foreign objects embedded in the cut. Place a DSD over the injury and bandage it. A knot should never be tied over the eye, as it causes pressure on the eyeball.

Blunt Injuries to the Eye Blunt injuries to the eye will usually cause hemorrhaging. Keep the person still and provide a dry, sterile dressing over the injury (it is preferable to cover both eyes to prevent any movement). Seek medical attention.

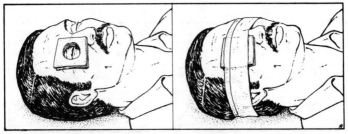

Figure 9 Embedded object in the eye. Apply gauze doughnut and cover the doughnut with a DSD. Apply roller bandage over both eyes.

Impaled Objects An impaled object is a stick, knife, glass, or similar object which protrudes from the wound. No attempt should be made to remove the impaled object. Cut off the remainder of the object several inches from the body if possible. Cut away any tight clothing.

Treatment With sterile gauze, pack heavily around the object, immobilizing it to the wound. Secure the gauze with a pressure bandage to control the bleeding (see Figure 10). Treat for shock and obtain immediate medical assistance.

Animal Bites The bite of any animal may be serious. The greatest danger is usually that of infection. It may be a puncture or an avulsion wound, depending upon the extent of the injury. An important concern with all animal bites is the possibility of rabies (see "Rabies," in Chapter 13).

Treatment If the wound is bleeding freely, control the bleeding. Wash the wound thoroughly with warm water and soap. Rinse with lots of water and apply a dry,

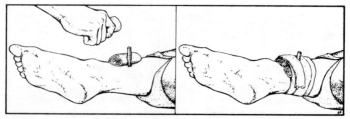

Figure 10 Impaled object. Apply thick gauze packs around wound and secure with elastic bandage.

sterile dressing. Refer the injury to a physician. Identify or capture the animal if this is possible without incurring any risk! Notify an animal control shelter.

Human Bites A severe human bite must be treated as a serious wound. These bites are common with young children and sometimes occur in adults. The wounds are heavily contaminated and there is always the danger of infection. Every human bite that breaks the skin should be seen by a physician.

Signs Teeth indentation, possible bruising of tissue, and breakage of the skin.

Treatment If the skin is broken, treat the wound as a puncture wound. Wash thoroughly with warm water and soap, and apply a mild antiseptic and a DSD. If the skin is not broken, treat as a bruise. Cleanse the area thoroughly and place an ice bag over the injury.

Splinters Splinters that are not deeply embedded are usually easy to remove. In the removal of a splinter, follow this procedure:

- Cleanse the area with soap and water.
- Sterilize a needle with disinfectant or by passing it through a flame.
- Allow the needle to cool and open the skin gently with the needle.
- Grasp the splinter with a pair of tweezers and gently work it out with the needle (see Figure 11).
- Treat the wound as a puncture wound.

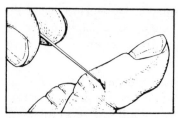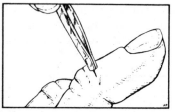

Figure 11 Technique to remove splinter with a needle and tweezers.

Splinters embedded under the nail should normally be referred to a physician. If medical help is unavailable, use the following procedure:

- Cleanse the nail with soap and water.
- Using a sharp blade, carefully pare the nail directly over the splinter, cutting through the nail.
- Using a sterile needle, work the splinter out from under the nail.

Splinters that go unremoved will usually become infected. If infection occurs:

- Apply hot compresses or soaks 15 to 20 minutes three to four times daily.
- Usually an abscess (pus) will form and the infection will "come to a head."
- Using the sterile needle, open the abscess and remove the splinter. Cleanse and apply a DSD.

Fishhook Often a deeply embedded fishhook cannot be removed the same way it entered without causing further injury. Application of an ice-cold compress to the area for a few moments will decrease the pain. In a wilderness situation one of the following two techniques may be considered in the removal of a fishhook:

Method A

- Remove the hook with the aid of a pair of pliers by advancing the fishhook in a curve so that the barbed tip exits through the skin.
- Clip off the barbed tip and withdraw the remainder of the hook the way it entered (see Figure 12a).
- Soak the injury in warm water; cleanse and treat it as a puncture wound.

Method B An alternate method of removing an embedded fishhook is to press down on the shank and pull the barb out with a quick jerk, as illustrated in Figure 12b. Although it appears more difficult than method A, this technique is less dangerous and causes less damage to the tissue.

Fingernail or Toenail Injuries

Contusion of the Nail With this type of injury the blood vessels are ruptured under the nail. Such an injury may be caused by hitting the fingernail with a hammer, pinching the fingers in a car door, or dropping a heavy object on the toe. The pressure of the blood under the nail may cause intense pain.

Signs Intense throbbing pain of the part. The area under the nail looks bright red at first and then turns black-and-blue.

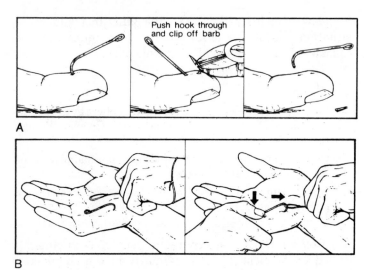

Figure 12 (a) Fishook removal. First ice area until numb, then advance hook, clip the barbed end of the hook, and remove remainder of shank. (b) Fishhook removal. First ice area until numb, then press down on shank and give quick jerk on line looped over the hook.

Treatment Apply a cold compress (ice bag) to the area to reduce the swelling. If medical help is unavailable, the pressure can be relieved by the following procedure:

- Cleanse the nail thoroughly with soap and water or a mild antiseptic.
- After unfolding a large paper clip, apply tape over one end. Heat the other end of the paper clip through a flame to red-hot.
- Apply the hot tip of the paper clip to the nail, reheating several times as necessary. *Note:* Apply the hot paper clip

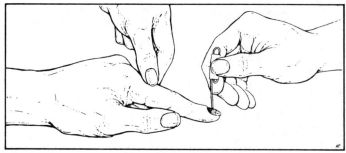

Figure 13 Nail injury. Technique used to relieve hematoma (collection of blood) from under the nail.

where the blood shows under the nail, as far toward the distal end of the finger or toe as possible.

- The hot end will burn through the nail, evacuating the blood and relieving the pain (see Figure 13).
- Cleanse the area with soap and water and apply a bandage over the nail.

Ingrown Toenail   Ingrown toenails may result from improperly trimming the nails or from jamming the toe. They are often painful and may become infected. Normally the nail should be trimmed straight across.

Signs   Redness, swelling, infection, and soreness at the edge of the nail.

Treatment   If the toe is jammed, use ice treatment to reduce swelling. If the toe becomes infected, apply hot compresses or soaks for 15 to 20 minutes, three to four times daily. If an abscess forms and medical help is unavailable, open the abscess with a sterile needle, cleanse, and apply a DSD. Notch the nail with a small v in the middle to permit a proper growth (see Figure 14).

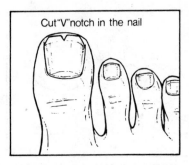

Figure 14 Proper technique for trimming an ingrown toenail.

Hangnail A hangnail infection may result from manicuring the nails too closely or from a trauma to the nail. The infection is usually limited to the end of the finger, at the edge of the nail.

Signs Soreness, redness, swelling, and infection present.

Treatment Apply hot compresses or soaks 15 to 20 minutes, three to four times daily. If an abscess forms, use a sterile needle to open and drain. Apply a DSD. Any infection extending up the finger or extremity needs medical attention.

Chapter 6
Dressing and Bandaging Wounds

The *dressing* refers to the material that is applied directly to the wound. Any material applied to an open wound should be sterile. The *bandage* is the material applied to the outside of the wound and covering the dressing. A dressing or bandage may serve several purposes when applied to a wound or an injury. It may be used to:

- Control bleeding by compression
- Prevent infection or contamination
- Provide pressure to reduce swelling
- Immobilize the area to reduce pain
- Provide support for the part

Dressings

A wound should first be covered with a dry, sterile gauze dressing or compress. This dry, sterile dressing is commonly referred to as a *DSD*. The dressing will absorb the bleeding and provide a cushion to the wound. It may be rolled gauze, a gauze pad, or a nonadhering dressing such as a Telfa or Adaptic sterile pad. Dressings can be made from lint-free cotton sheets or a similar cloth. Launder, iron, and cut the material into strips 2 to 6 inches in width and approximately 36 inches in length. Roll the strips of cloth and place them in a plastic wrap to ensure cleanliness.

Bandages

Bandages are usually classified as *roller, triangular,* or *adhesive.*

- *Roller bandages* are rolled strips of cloth or an elastic bandage.
- *Triangular bandages* are three-cornered bandages of approximately 60 inches across the base. They may be folded into a bandage called a *cravat.*
- *Adhesive bandages* are combinations of dressings and bandages such as Band-Aid adhesive bandages and butterfly strips.

Any bandage applied to an open wound must be firm enough to control the bleeding. Care must be exercised in applying the bandage. If it is too tight, it may cut off circulation to the area beyond the wound. If swelling, numbness, or blueness occurs beyond the injury, the bandage should be loosened and reapplied. If the initial wraps are applied securely but not tightly, loss of circulation should not occur. *Caution:* Do not remove the dressing if it is necessary to loosen and reapply the bandage. Removing the dressing may cause the wound to bleed.

Elastic Multipurpose Bandage   The 4-inch elastic bandage is the ideal size for many injuries and a must for any first-aid kit. This bandage is easy to apply and stays in place better than most other bandages. It can be used as a support bandage for sprains, strains, and dislocations; it can be applied over a sterile dressing as a pressure bandage, or lightly secured over sterile dressings for burns; it may also be used to immobilize fractures.

Triangular Bandage   The triangular bandage, which may be folded as a cravat (two or three folds), is another multipurpose bandage (see Figure 1). A cravat bandage can be used to secure a pressure bandage, as a constricting band, or as a tourniquet. Like a triangular bandage, it may also be used as a sling, or to cover areas of the body which are difficult to bandage. Two triangular bandages can be made from a square yard of muslin or similar material by cutting diagonally.

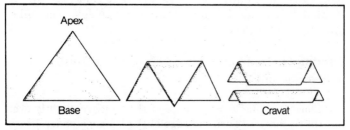

Figure 1   Folding the triangular bandage to make a cravat bandage.

Adhesive Bandage   The adhesive bandage is a prepackaged sterile bandage that can be purchased in various sizes. Examples of these bandages are Band-Aid adhesive bandages, butterfly strips, and adhesive coverlet bandages.

General Guidelines for Bandage Application

Following is a general description of the application of the triangular and cravat bandages to various parts of the body. An alternative technique using the elastic or roller bandage is also suggested. Some prefer this method of bandaging. The type of bandage selected usually depends upon the place of the injury and the materials available at the time. The most important consideration in the application of any bandage is that it should be firmly applied and well secured over the wound or the injured part. The more you practice these bandaging techniques the more adept you will become in their application.

The *square knot* should be used to secure most bandages. It is simple to tie and easy to release. The tie is made by taking the ends of the bandage, left over right, and then right over left.

Bandage to Head or Scalp   This bandage is used to hold a dressing on the forehead or the scalp.

- Place the middle of the base of the bandage slightly over the eyebrows. Turn the edge of the bandage under 1 inch as a hem for added strength.

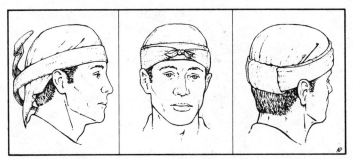

Figure 2 Applying a triangular bandage as a head dressing.

- Allow the point or tail of the bandage to drop over the back of the head.
- Cross the ends over the point and make a single tie at the base of the skull. Tuck the point securely into the tie and pull taut.
- Bring the ends of the bandage around to the forehead and secure the tie (see Figure 2).

Pressure Bandage to Head or Scalp This bandage is used to control severe bleeding from the scalp. Apply the dressing over the wound and use the cravat to cover.

- Place the midpoint of the cravat bandage over the dressing.
- Make one tie around the base of the skull to hold firmly in place.
- Secure the bandage by tying the ends of the cravat over the wound (see Figure 3).

Note: Do not tie the knot over the wound if an embedded object is in the wound.

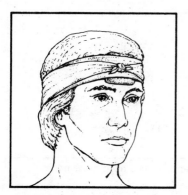

Figure 3 Applying a cravat pressure bandage to a scalp wound.

Alternative Method Place the dressing over the wound. Use the gauze or elastic bandage by wrapping around the head several times. Secure with the metal clip or a piece of tape.

Bandage to Head, Ear, or Chin This bandage is used to hold a dressing in place on the side of the head, ear, or chin.

- Place the cravat over the dressing at the midpoint.
- Bring it under the chin and over the top of the skull.
- Cross the bandage on the opposite side of the head and bring across the forehead and the back of the head.
- The ends of the bandage should meet over the primary turn of the cravat. Secure with a square knot (see Figure 4).

Alternative Method Apply a dressing to the wound and secure with an elastic bandage. The elastic bandage will easily conform to the head if applied at an angle over the forehead and at the base of the skull.

Figure 4 Applying a pressure bandage to the side of the head.

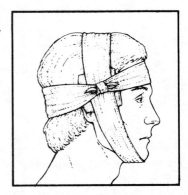

Bandage to Eye   This bandage is used to hold a dressing over an injured eye.

- Place a strip of cloth (2 inches in width and 15 inches in length) at an angle over the top of the head and drooping over the uninjured eye, near the nose.
- Bring the cravat over the dressing and make one tie at the base of the skull. Start the cravat slightly off center so that the final tie is not over the eye.
- Bring the ends of the bandage around the forehead and secure.
- Bring the strip of cloth to the top of the head and tie. This will pull the cravat up from the uninjured eye (see Figure 5).

Alternative Method   Apply a dressing over the injured eye. Wrap a gauze or elastic bandage lightly around the head at an angle to allow sight out of the uninjured eye. Another method is to apply an eye patch and secure it with two strips of adhesive tape.

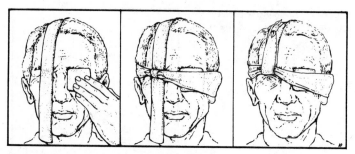

Figure 5 The steps in applying a bandage to cover the eye.

Note: If both eyes are injured, cover each eye with a light compress and bring the cravat, gauze roller, or elastic bandage directly over the eyes and around the skull.

Bandage to Shoulder The triangular bandage is used to hold a dressing on wounds and burns to the shoulder.

- Place the point of the triangular bandage over the shoulder.
- Roll the point into a strip of cloth or a cravat bandage and tie across the chest and under the opposite arm (do not tie knot under the armpit).
- Fold the base of the bandage under to assist in holding the dressing in place.
- Bring the ends of the bandage under the arm to completely enclose the area under the arm. Secure the bandage over the fold.
- Readjust the strip of cloth or cravat bandage as necessary (see Figure 6).

Alternative Method If the wound is not above the shoulder, apply a dressing and cover it with a closed-

Figure 6 Applying the triangular bandage to the shoulder.

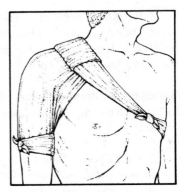

spiral elastic bandage (see alternative method under "Bandage to Hip," below).

Bandage to Hip To apply the triangular bandage to the hip, use the same basic technique indicated for the shoulder (see Figure 7). Secure the point of the bandage at the waist in a belt or a similar tie. Wrap the ends around the leg and secure.

Figure 7 Applying the triangular bandage to the hip.

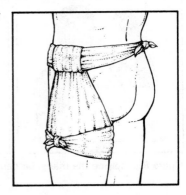

Alternative Method The use of the closed-spiral elastic bandage over a dressing is an excellent method of holding a dressing in place on wounds to the hip. Start the wrap low and wrap to the higher part of the leg.

Bandage to Chest or Back Use the triangular bandage to hold a dressing on wounds, especially burns of the chest or back.

- Place the point of the bandage over the shoulder. The base of the bandage will cover the chest or back.
- Hem the bandage and tie around the front or back, leaving one end of the bandage longer than the other.
- Tie the point to the long end of the first tie.
- Adjust the bandage at the shoulder and under the arm so that it is securely in place (see Figure 8).

Sling The triangular bandage may be used as a sling for support of injuries to the arm or shoulder (Figure 9).

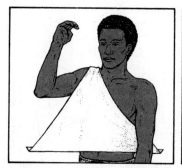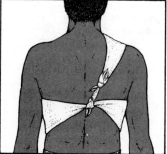

Figure 8 Applying the triangular bandage to the chest.

- Place the triangular bandage on the chest so that the point is at the elbow of the injured arm.
- One end of the bandage will drape over the shoulder, opposite the injury.
- Place the injured arm on the bandage and bring the other end of the bandage over the arm.
- Make the tie around the neck, elevating the arm slightly above the horizontal position.
- Tie a knot or pin the bandage at the point to cradle the elbow.
- Adjust the bandage so that the fingers will cup over the edge of the sling.
- To eliminate movement, tie one or two cravats over the injured arm (slightly above the elbow and at the shoulder) and secure under the opposite arm.

Alternative Method

- Elastic wrap. Place the arm on the chest, slightly above the horizontal position. Wrap an elastic bandage alternately around the chest and over the opposite shoulder and

Figure 9 Using the triangular bandage as a sling.

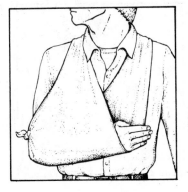

back, enclosing the arm from the elbow to the wrist. If the shoulder is injured, provide additional wrap between shoulder and elbow. (See bandages described under "Fracture of the Ribs" in Chapter 7.)

- A loose-knit shirt or bulky sweater makes an ideal sling. Bring the bottom of the shirt or sweater over the arm, supporting it as you would with a triangular bandage. Tie or secure the extra material in a single knot at the back so the bottom of the shirt or sweater will cradle the arm (see Figure 10).

- Long-tailed shirt. A long-tailed or loose-fitting shirt will also make an excellent sling. First unbutton several of the bottom buttons. Support the injured arm by bringing the tail of the shirt over the arm and the elbow. Bring the other shirttail around the back and over the opposite shoulder. Make the tie where the shirttail ends meet, supporting the arm slightly above the horizontal position.

Note: All of these methods will securely immobilize the arm to the chest.

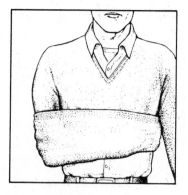

Figure 10 Using a sweater as a sling.

Bandage to Hand or Foot Use the triangular bandage to cover wounds or burns to the hand or foot.

- Place the bandage so that the point is above the fingers or toes.
- Bring the point of the bandage over the fingers or toes so that it completely covers the part.
- Tuck the excess material in close to the hand or foot.
- Bring the ends across the hand or foot, and secure by tying around the wrist or ankle (see Figure 11).

Bandage to Elbow or Knee The cravat bandage is used to hold a dressing around the elbow or knee.

- Bend the joint (elbow or knee) and place the center of the cravat at the point of the elbow or front of the knee.
- Bring the ends across each other; the top end of the cravat crosses below the joint and the bottom end crosses above the joint.
- Overlap the bandage with a closed-spiral turn (both above and below).
- Secure the ends of the cravat by tying it over the wound.

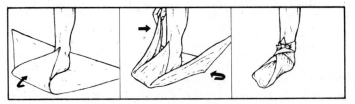

Figure 11 Applying the triangular bandage to the foot.

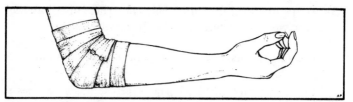

Figure 12 An elastic bandage used to secure a dressing to the elbow.

Alternative Method The elastic bandage is ideally suited to hold a dressing about an injury to the elbow or knee joint. Apply the spiral bandage over the dressing while the joint is in a flexed position. Secure with a metal clip or tape (see Figure 12).

Bandage to Arm or Leg The cravat bandage may be applied to hold a dressing in place on the arm or leg. It is applied as follows for bandages for the elbow or knee:

- Place the center of the cravat over the dressing around the arm or leg.
- Bring the bandage ends around the arm or leg, overlapping approximately one-third of the previous wrap. One end of the cravat wraps high, and the other low.
- Bring the ends of the bandage back to the center to make the tie (see Figure 13).

Alternative Method Apply an elastic or roller bandage using a one-third overlapping spiral turn to securely hold the dressing in place. This bandage is easier to apply and will stay in place much better than the cravat (see below, "Closed-Spiral Bandage").

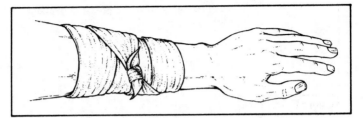

Figure 13 Applying the cravat bandage to the forearm.

Bandage to Hand A figure-eight bandage is used to cover a dressing to the palm or the back of the hand.

- Place a dressing over the wound and use a cravat, gauze, or elastic bandage to cover.
- Start the wraps below the tips of the fingers, slightly overlapping each preceding wrap.
- Allowing the thumb to stay exposed, bring the wrap to the wrist and secure it (see Figure 14).

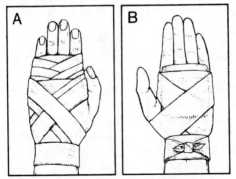

Figure 14 Using (a) an elastic bandage and (b) a gauze roller bandage as a figure eight to secure a dressing to the hand.

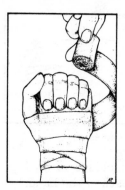

Figure 15 Applying a pressure bandage of the hand.

Pressure Bandage to Hand This bandage is used to control severe bleeding to the palm of the hand.

- Place a large dressing or folded compress in the hand; have the victim squeeze the compress by clenching the fist.
- Apply a gauze or elastic bandage, encircling the fist with overlapping wraps around the fingers, thumb, and wrist (see Figure 15).

Closed-Spiral Bandage This type of dressing is recommended for burns or as a bandage covering wounds to the extremities. The closed-spiral dressing is applied directly to the wound. The new improved gauze is especially easy to apply as it stretches and clings to the skin. If the spiral bandage is used, apply directly over the dressing.

- Anchor the dressing or bandage by making several turns below the injury.

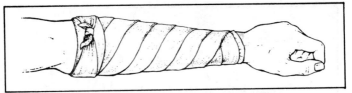

Figure 16 Applying a closed-spiral bandage to the forearm.

- Bring the dressing around the entire extremity, overlapping by one-third of the dressing with each circular turn.
- If the dressing is applied to burns, it is often necessary to overlap the bandage to keep the air out of the injury.
- The dressing may be secured with tape or by splitting the bandage and tying a single knot at the tear. Bring the ends around the extremity and tie.
- Bandages may be secured with a clip or tape (see Figure 16).

Open-Spiral Bandage   An open-spiral bandage is used to cover a dressing but still allow the wound to breathe. If there is a danger of the wound becoming contaminated by dust, this bandage should not be used.

- Anchor the bandage by making several turns around the dressing.
- Make circular turns around the extremity with an open area between the turns. Secure bandage with a clip or tie (see Figure 17).

Alternative Method   Apply sterile dressing and secure at the ends with adhesive tape (see Chapter 5, Figure 6).

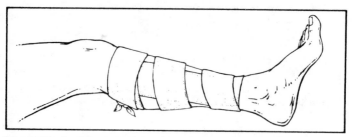

Figure 17 Applying an open-spiral bandage.

Butterfly Strip   This bandage is used to close a severe
cut once the bleeding has been controlled. The butterfly
may be a self-adhering bandage or improvised from
adhesive tape.

- Make several butterfly strips by cutting to the appropriate
  size from adhesive tape.
- Fold the middle of the adhesive part of the tape together.
- Light a match and singe the folded tape, which will pass
  directly over the wound.

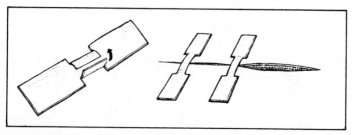

Figure 18   Making and applying butterfly strips to close an open
wound.

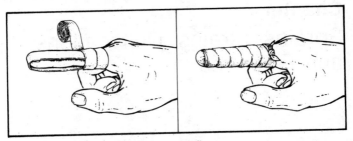

Figure 19 Applying a bandage to the finger.

- Stick one end of the tape to the skin and bring the open parts of the wound together. Press the other end of the butterfly firmly to the skin to close the wound. Use as many butterfly strips as necessary to close the entire wound (see Figure 18).
- Cover with a sterile dressing and bandage.

Bandage to Finger or Toe   To bandage cuts or injuries to the fingers or toes where the adhesive bandage will not suffice, use the spiral turn technique. Use 1-inch sterile gauze and secure with adhesive tape (see Figure 19).

Chapter 7

Sprains, Strains, Dislocations, and Fractures

Sprains, strains, and dislocations are injuries that occur to the muscles or to the tendons and ligaments around the joints. A dislocation involves the displacement of the bone ends from the joint, and a fracture is any break in the bone itself. A sprain, dislocation, and fracture may be present in the same injury, depending upon its location and severity. The general treatment for all muscular injuries is essentially the same. These are the injuries most frequently incurred along the trail or during any vigorous activity.

Sprains

A sprain is an injury to the joint, usually the ankle or the knee, involving the ligaments. Some muscle damage may occur. The joint has been twisted or stretched beyond its normal limits, causing a tearing of the various tissues. Sprains will vary in severity from a minor twisting of the part to serious tissue damage of the joint with an accompanying fracture.

Signs Pain will vary with the degree of severity and increase with any movement or weight bearing on the part. There may be considerable soreness, swelling, and edema of the joint. Discoloration may be present due to internal bleeding in the joint.

Treatment Apply a cold compress or ice bag to the area. Elevate the part 18 inches and anchor the compress securely with a light pressure bandage. The cold compress should be applied for 30 minutes, removed, and then reapplied. Cold applications are used for a period of 6 to 48 hours depending upon the severity of the injury. After removing the cold compress, apply a pressure bandage, elevate above heart level, and rest for 30 minutes (see Figures 1 and 2). Repeat this alternating technique of 30 minutes of cold and 30 minutes of rest as long as swelling persists. In sprains that are extremely severe and involve rapid swelling, the cold compress should be maintained for longer periods of time. Refer the person to a hospital for further evaluation. *Caution:* Do not apply ice directly to the part or immerse in ice water. A thin cloth or light

Figure 1 Use a figure-eight wrap with a 4-inch elastic bandage to support a sprain of the ankle.

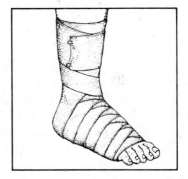

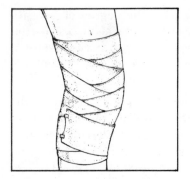

Figure 2 Use a figure-eight wrap with a 4-inch elastic bandage to support a sprain of the knee.

plastic film must be placed between the injury and the ice to prevent frostbite or freezing of the tissue. Heat therapy will be helpful a day or two after the cold treatment has been completed. Apply heat with warm towels or whirlpool therapy for 20 minutes, three or four times a day. *Note:* Cold constricts the blood vessels and decreases circulation, lessening bleeding and swelling. Later, the application of heat will increase the circulation and aid in the healing process.

Strains

Strains are distinguished from sprains in that a strain involves the tearing of the muscle or the muscle-tendon unit. This occurs from overexertion or the overstretching of the muscle. There is often an associated injury to the tendon which attaches the muscle to the bone. The most common injuries occur to the large muscles of the back and the upper and lower leg.

Signs The pain varies with the severity. There may be considerable swelling, edema, discoloration, stiffness, and firmness in the area injured. Any movement intensifies the pain.

Treatment The treatment is essentially the same as for the sprain. Apply cold compresses; provide rest, elevation if possible, and limited activity. Any severe strain should be seen by a physician. *Caution:* Do not apply heat to a strain during the first 24 to 48 hours, as it will increase the swelling and fluid in the tissue, compounding the injury. Refer to follow-up therapy for sprains.

Charley Horse A *charley horse* is a severely pulled or bruised muscle of the thigh (contusion of the quadriceps muscle).[1] Intramuscular bleeding occurs from the torn muscle fibers.

Signs Intense pain over area, especially on movement. Swelling, stiffness, discoloration (ecchymosis and hematoma formation), and muscle spasm may develop.

Treatment Apply ice therapy as in a severe strain, pressure bandage, and elevation for 24 to 36 hours. Seek medical attention.

Minor Muscular Problems General muscular aches and discomforts, muscle spasm, stiff neck, and muscle fatigue are often caused by fatigue and overexertion. If rest or

---

[1] *Standard Nomenclature of Athletic Injuries,* American Medical Association, 535 North Dearborn Street, Chicago, IL 60610.

treatment is not provided, a more extensive injury may occur.

Treatment The application of warm, moist towels to the area, or taking a hot shower or bath for 30 minutes will alleviate soreness, relieve pain, and improve circulation. Repeat this treatment as necessary. Rest and fluids by mouth are recommended.

Tendonitis Tendonitis is an inflammation of the tendons and their attachments to the muscles and bones. A strain of the Achilles tendon is an example.

Signs Pain in the area, aggravated by movement. Possible swelling and inflammation.

Treatment Apply cold to the area. Apply cold pack or rub an ice cube over the area for 15 to 20 minutes three or four times daily. After each cold treatment, strap or support the area with a 4-inch elastic bandage. Limit activity for 1 to 3 weeks. Heat may be applied after the condition improves. If the condition does not improve, refer to a physician.

Bursitis Bursitis is an inflammation of the bursa in the joint area. A bursa is a small sac located under the tendon or muscle which cushions movement. Inflammation is often caused by excessive movement or pressure of the joint. *Tennis elbow* and *housemaid's knee* are examples.

Signs Similar to tendonitis.

Treatment See preceding section, "Tendonitis." Support the part with elastic bandage during any activity.

Dislocations

A dislocation occurs in the joints when the bone is forced out of its socket or otherwise displaced from its normal location. There will be muscle, tendon, ligament, and capsular damage to the joint. Fractures of the associated bones may occur, with the possibility of nerve and blood vessel damage. The reduction of a dislocation should be left to a physician; however, in a *remote* wilderness setting the reduction of certain types of dislocations may be considered.

Signs Usually there will be considerable pain and swelling, especially upon any movement of the joint. Loss of movement, numbness, and paralysis may be present. There will be a marked deformity or a distinct displacement of the bone at the joint.

Treatment Normal treatment for all dislocations includes cold compress and pressure bandage to immobilize the injury. Treat most joint injuries in the way you would a fracture. Refer to a hospital. The physician will usually x-ray to rule out possible fracture prior to the reduction of any dislocation. In remote areas reductions of dislocated jaws, fingers, and shoulders have been performed successfully by nonmedical people.

Jaw A person may dislocate the jaw by yawning. Normally the dislocated jaw is not difficult to reduce. Insert thumbs, well padded with gauze, over the back of the lower molars. Cup the fingers under the person's chin and firmly press downward and backward. Lift the chin upward as the back portion of the jaw begins to move.

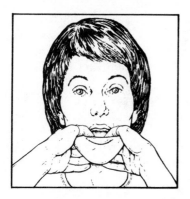

Figure 3 Reducing a dislocation of the jaw.

Quickly slip the fingers to the side of the jawbone as the jaw snaps into position (see Figure 3).

Fingers Dislocation of the fingers usually occurs in the second joint. Reduction is accomplished by pulling firmly on the finger beyond the dislocated joint (see Figure 4). After the dislocation is reduced, apply a cold compress to the area. Wrap the injured finger securely to the adjacent finger to immobilize the injury. No attempt should be made to reduce a dislocated thumb as it usually involves a fracture and tendon damage. Apply a cold compress,

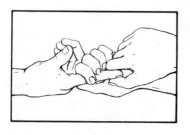

Figure 4 Reducing a dislocation of the finger.

immobilize, and elevate. Do not use the injured hand. This injury should be seen by a physician who specializes in the hand.

Shoulder   Most shoulders are dislocated by a severe force driving the arm backward and displacing the head of the humerus (upper arm bone) from the shoulder socket. This usually dislocates the shoulder forward. A person who extends the hand to break a fall may dislocate the shoulder backward. In either case there is always a tear of the shoulder capsule and severe ligament damage. A comparison of both shoulders helps in deciding whether there is a dislocation present. If there is considerable pain and muscle spasm in the shoulder area, make no attempt to reduce the dislocation. The *key* in the reduction of a shoulder dislocation is to be as gentle and careful as possible when applying traction to the part. Force is *not* required, nor should it be used. Reduce only a forward dislocation.

Treatment for Shoulder Dislocation

Gravity Reduction   If you are attempting a shoulder dislocation reduction, allow gravity to reduce the dislocation. Place the person in a prone position (face down) on a table or something similar in height. Strap a 5-pound weight to the wrist and allow it to hang over the side. Keep the person as relaxed as possible. After a few minutes the head of the humerus may gently slip back into the proper position (see Figure 5). Another technique is to strap a bucket to the wrist and gradually add sand or water to the bucket. Do not have the victim grasp the bucket with the hand, as this will create muscle tension.

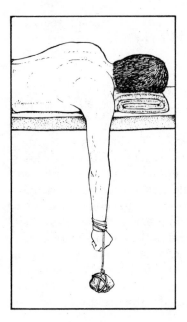

Figure 5 The gravity reduction method for reducing a dislocation of the shoulder.

Other dislocations which should be treated, but not reduced, include the hip, ankle, wrist, elbow, and knee.

Hip The hip dislocation is somewhat similar to the shoulder. It involves the large muscles and ligaments of the thigh and pelvic area and is usually sustained in serious automobile accidents. Often there are associated injuries to the femur or pelvis. Reduction should be done only by a physician. Immobilize the person on a spinal board in a supine position with the leg slightly elevated. Support the leg with a rolled blanket or pillows, and secure it to the spinal board to prevent movement.

This person should be transported by ambulance to the hospital. *Treat for shock.*

Ankle, Wrist, Elbow, and Knee   No attempt should be made to reduce a dislocation of the ankle, wrist, elbow, or knee. There is often a fracture accompanying the dislocation. These dislocations should be immobilized and splinted, if necessary, in their present position. Apply a cold compress to the area.

Kneecap   A dislocation of the kneecap (patella) may occur in a fall or result from a severe blow to the knee. The kneecap is usually displaced to the outside and below the knee. The pain is generally severe, and the leg is in a flexed position. Apply a cold compress and immobilize the leg in its present position. If the pain is not too severe, a gradual straightening of the leg may cause the kneecap to slip back into proper position, reducing the dislocation. Immobilize the leg in this position by splinting below the kneecap (see Figure 6). Transport the person to the hospital.

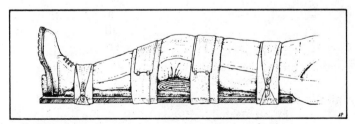

Figure 6   Splinting a dislocation of the patella (kneecap).

Fractures

A fracture is a break in the bone and may vary from the simple to the complex. Fractures are classified as open or closed. In an open fracture an associated wound must be treated, as the bone has penetrated through the skin. This wound must be cared for initially by the application of a pressure bandage; next, as in all fractures, the part must be carefully immobilized.

Signs Pain, tenderness, swelling, and loss of function at the site. Possible deformity or shortening of the extremity with later discoloration. The person may hear or feel something snap during the mishap, or feel the bones grate against each other.

Treatment Treatment consists of immobilization, controlling the bleeding in an open wound, reduction of pain, splinting, and providing proper transportation. Individuals with fractures of the upper extremities, shoulders, ribs, and collarbones can walk under most circumstances. Individuals with fractures of the lower extremities, spinal column, and hip and those individuals with severe head injuries must be carried. Great resourcefulness and ingenuity, and numerous assistants are often required to evacuate individuals with these types of injuries. Primary considerations for individuals with spinal injuries are to make them immobile and comfortable, and to obtain medical rescue assistance.

Splinting Different materials are discussed here to demonstrate the available options in applying splints to various parts of the body. One type of splint is not necessarily better than the other. If you decide to splint you should use the best, most lightweight materials available.

The purpose of the splint is to relieve pain and prevent any additional movement of the fractured bone, especially if the person is to be moved. The decision of whether or not to splint most fractures depends upon the immediacy of emergency aid, materials available with which to splint, and the method of transportation. If an ambulance is deemed necessary and readily available, keep the person immobile and quiet with the extremity and the fracture still. Do not splint, as the emergency medical technician (EMT) or paramedic will do so upon arrival. With respect to simple closed fractures of the fingers, arms, collarbone, etc., it may be appropriate to splint and transport to a hospital by automobile. In remote settings the decision to splint depends upon the nature of the injury, time factor, materials available, necessity of moving the person, and method of evacuation. Usually splinting is indicated with the exception of spinal injuries, in which case professional medical help to evacuate is mandatory. If the individual must be moved, splint.

Materials selected for most splinting should be lightweight, e.g., corrugated cardboard, wire mesh, shingles padded with cloth or foam rubber, magazines, rolled-up newspapers, or pillows. Inflatable splints are convenient; however, these splints need careful attention due to the possibility of overinflation and consequent restriction of circulation. Splinting of one leg to the other with a blanket inserted between and a firm object to the outside is acceptable. Splints for the back and hip require complete immobilization. Great care must be exercised with this type of injury. Listed below are some general guidelines for splinting:

- Always cut away the clothing from any suspected fracture.
- Cover any wound with a sterile dressing prior to splinting.
- Do not attempt to push any broken bones back or set a fracture (splint "as is" if possible).
- Immobilize the joint above and below the fracture.
- Pad the splint well to equalize pressure and to fit the contour of the extremity.
- Affix the splint to the flat surface of the extremity.
- A gentle traction of the extremity may be necessary in some cases exhibiting deformity to properly affix the splint (do not release pressure until splint is secure).
- Prepare all materials to proper size prior to splinting.
- Splints can be held in place with strips of cloth or cravat or roller bandages.
- Do not move the person prior to splinting and transporting.
- The splint should be secure. It may be necessary to loosen and reapply if the person complains of numbness, tingling sensation, or inability to move fingers or toes.
- If in doubt whether or not a fracture exists, splint.
- *Treat for shock.*

Fracture of the Skull A blow to the skull may cause damage to the blood vessels which supply the brain or its coverings. Any injury of this nature must be considered serious. A skull fracture must be suspected in any unconscious or semiconscious person who has sustained a head injury. Indicators include bleeding or oozing of watery fluid from the ears or nose, unequal size of the pupils, ringing of the ears, and intense headache, if conscious. In providing treatment, keep the person absolutely still. *Do not move.* Ensure an open airway. Control any external bleeding with direct-pressure bandage and treat the person for shock. Do not administer any fluids. Arrange for an ambulance. A stretcher should be used to transport a person who has suffered a skull fracture.

The 24-Hour Period Following a Head Injury   A person who has sustained a head injury should be closely observed for possible aftereffects for the next 24 hours. There may be no evidence of a serious head injury present during the initial examination. The victim should be awakened every 2 hours during this period to check his or her condition. If any of the following signs or symptoms develop, *immediately* contact a physician or the hospital emergency department.

- Increased drowsiness; difficulty in arousing the person
- Irritability or marked restlessness
- Confusion, slurred speech, or double vision
- One pupil appearing larger than the other
- Severe and/or persistent vomiting
- Drainage of blood or clear fluid from ear or nose
- Convulsions or loss of strength in the extremities
- Stiffness of the neck and/or temperature of over 100°F

Note: It is important that the victim of a head injury should drink no alcoholic beverages and eat only light meals during the following 24 to 48 hours. Victims should take only the medication that has been prescribed for them.

Fracture of the Nose A nose fracture is commonly caused by a severe blow to the nose. The nose is usually pushed to one side of the face. The victim often experiences intense pain, and there will probably be bleeding from the nose. If medical help is available, do not attempt to straighten the nose. Cleanse any external wound with soap and water and apply a soft protective compress. Application of a cold compress to the area will minimize the swelling. Treat any nasal bleeding (see "Nosebleed" in Chapter 5). If medical help is available within a week or so, do the following: Apply the soft protective compress and advise the victim to breathe through the mouth. Normally you should not splint a fracture of the nose. Seek medical advice. *Note:* If medical help is unavailable, the nose can usually be pushed back into proper position by grasping the nose with the thumb and forefinger and moving it to its original position.

Fracture of the Jaw Little can be done to treat a fracture of the *upper jaw*. The severity of the blow causing the fracture may indicate a skull fracture. Keep the victim still and hospitalize as soon as possible. Fractures of the *lower jaw* are usually painful, with an obvious displacement. The victim usually has difficulty in opening or moving the jaw. There may be an uneven alignment of the teeth and a drooling of saliva or blood from the mouth. If medical help is available, do not treat. It is not advisable that this fracture be bandaged, as the airway needs to be kept open at all times. To relieve pain, have the victim support the lower jaw with a hand so that the lower teeth rest against the upper. Obtain medical assistance.

Note: Extended travel time to a hospital may make it necessary to support the jaw with a bandage. First close the jaw gently so that the lower teeth rest against the upper. Apply a four-tail bandage with a 4-inch strip of cloth (see Figure 7). If the person becomes nauseous, loosen the bandage so the victim can vomit. Support the lower jaw until the vomiting ceases. Reapply the bandage and transport the person to a hospital.

Fracture of the Neck and/or Back Be extremely hesitant to move an individual who has injured the neck or back if spinal injury is suspected. Any fracture involving the spine is a serious medical problem, and emergency medical service should be obtained. Do not move the victim unless absolutely necessary. No attempt should

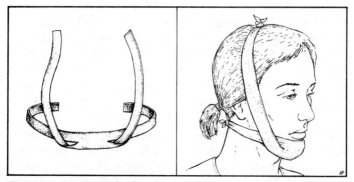

Figure 7 Support bandage for lower jaw if medical assistance not available.

be made to splint this type of injury without adequate knowledge, materials, and personnel. Any movement may compound the injury. If conscious, the person can usually tell you of pain along the spinal column. (If the neck is broken, the victim may not be able to move any fingers; if the back is broken, the person may not be able to move any toes.) If the victim is unconscious, you may be able to determine the injury by pricking the hand or foot with a pin. If the part moves, the person is not paralyzed. You may also check the spinal column by running your fingers along the vertebrae for obvious alignment problems. The victim of a spinal column injury should be completely immobilized with blankets or bulky clothing. Proper medical assistance and an ambulance should be obtained. In diving-board accidents a special problem exists, as the person needs to be removed from the water. Prior to removal from the water, insert a backboard or surfboard under the victim and stabilize the neck. Immobilize the injured person in this position and obtain an ambulance.

Note: If it is deemed necessary to move a person who has suffered an injury to the spinal column, you should have at least four people to assist. Furthermore, it is recommended that practice be performed on another member of the group several times prior to the move (see Chapter 15, "Carries and Short-Distance Transfers").

Fracture of the Neck A victim who has suffered a neck injury must be transported on a firm surface, generally lying on the back. If not already supine, the person must be carefully turned to this positon, but only if proper help is available. If the victim's head is in a twisted position, splint as is unless an airway obstruction exists. The neck should be straightened only to aid in opening the airway if breathing is not present.

The injured person should not be moved until the backboard is prepared, so that he or she will be moved one time only. Firm support and gentle traction to the head must be maintained as the victim is moved. Immobilize the head with heavy rolled cloths or towels placed on each side of the head (see Figure 8). To move the victim onto a backboard using traction applied to the head, refer to Chapter 15, "Carries and Short-Distance Transfers." Once placed on the backboard, the person must be securely immobilized. Elevate the lower end (foot) of the backboard about 12 inches to shock posi-

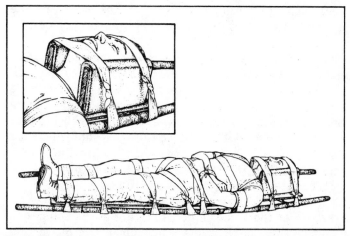

Figure 8 Extreme care must be exercised in immobilizing a person with a fracture of the neck. Inset demonstrates padding of the head and neck.

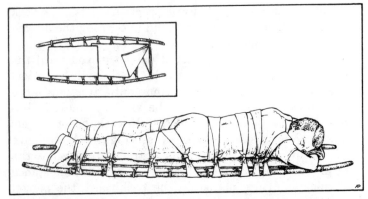

Figure 9 Transporting an injured person lying in a prone position. Inset depicts stretcher made from sticks, rope, and insulated padding.

tion. *Note:* If the victim is lying on the side, affix the splint to the person in this position prior to the turn.

Fracture of the Back The generally recommended treatment for a person who has suffered a fracture of the back is to transport in the position in which the victim is found. If the person is in a prone position, use the same gentle procedures in transferring onto the backboard that would be employed if the person were in a supine position (see Figure 9). In transporting the victim lying in a supine position, insert padding, such as a towel, to the spineboard to support the small of the back.

Fracture of the Collarbone Fracture of the collarbone (clavicle) commonly results from falls, direct blows, and especially from contact sports. The victim usually knows that the collarbone is broken and has difficulty raising the arm. The shoulder may droop on the affected side, and the victim will tend to hold the arm at the elbow for support. In palpating the collarbone you can usually feel a slight depression of the bone. Normally this injury is not considered serious. Two methods may be employed to support a broken collarbone. In the conventional method, a sling is applied to the arm of the affected side so it is elevated slightly above the horizontal position (see Figure 10). A towel or similar padding should be placed between the arm and the chest. Use two cravat bandages or ties to immobilize the arm to the side. An ice bag may be placed over the broken collarbone to reduce the swelling. The arm can also be supported in this position with an elastic wrap, or by merely pulling a bulky sweater or knit shirt over the arm and securing it with a tie (see Chapter 6, Figure 10).

Ideally, when medical help is not available, support a broken collarbone by using a 4-inch elastic *figure-eight* wrap around the shoulders, behind the neck, and under the arms. This strapping technique has the effect of pulling the shoulders back and pushing the neck and

Figure 10   A temporary support bandage for a fracture of the collarbone.

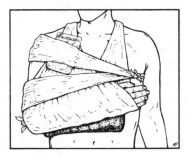

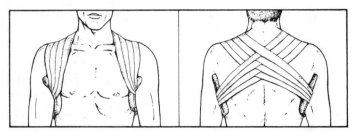

Figure 11 Using an elastic support bandage for a fracture of the collarbone.

head forward. It will provide support for the collarbone, placing it in its original position. When one is treating a fracture of the collarbone with this technique, the use of two elastic bandages for maximum support is recommended (see Figure 11).

Fracture of the Ribs Fracture of the ribs is caused by a direct blow or a compression injury, such as the jamming of the chest into the steering wheel during an automobile accident. The most commonly fractured ribs are the fifth through the tenth. Ribs 1 to 4 are seldom fractured, as they are well protected by the scapula and the clavicle. The lower two ribs (11 and 12) are floating ribs, having greater freedom of movement, and are not likely to be fractured. The victim will have localized pain at the site of the fracture and may experience intense pain during respiration. The person can usually pinpoint the exact location of the injury. There may or may not be a depression of the chest cavity. The victim usually prefers to stay still and immobilize the fracture by holding a hand over the injured area. If the victim coughs up bright

Figure 12 Using an elastic bandage to immobilize a fracture of the ribs.

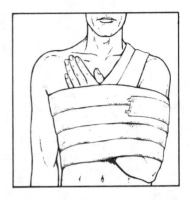

red, frothy blood, the fractured rib probably has also injured the lung. In the treatment of fractured ribs, they are not strapped unless the victim is extremely uncomfortable. *Do not strap* the ribs if there has been an injury to the lungs. The binding of the chest cavity will decrease respiration, compress the lungs, and increase the likelihood of a secondary infection (pneumonia). If it is deemed necessary to immobilize the chest cavity (no lung injury), use an elastic or wide-swathe bandage. Strap firmly (not tightly) around the chest, immobilizing the arm on the side of the fracture (see Figure 12). If ribs are fractured on both sides, immobilize both arms across the chest with a similar bandage. (The reason for immobilizing the rib cage is to limit painful movement if it is necessary for the victim to walk a long distance.)

Fracture of the Hand If an injured hand has been fractured and is to be splinted, always place the hand in a functional position. To achieve this position for the

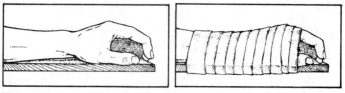

Figure 13 Immobilize a fracture of the hand in a functional position.

hand, place a roll of gauze or padding in the palm. Immobilize the hand with a padded splint, using an elastic or swathe bandage (see Figure 13).

Fracture of the Finger The finger should be immobilized in a slightly bent position. The finger may be strapped to an adjacent finger for support. Applying a slightly curved plastic or padded aluminum splint is an ideal method of splinting a fractured finger. Do not use a straight-edge splint such as a tongue depressor, as the finger should be splinted in a functional position (see Figure 14).

Fracture of Lower Arm and Wrist The most common fractures of the forearm (radius and ulna) occur at the wrist. This type of fracture may involve either or both

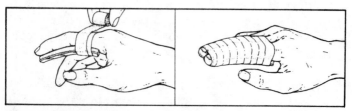

Figure 14 Immobilize a fractured finger in a functional position.

wrist bones. The fractured wrist should be immobilized with two padded splints to the flat part of the lower arm. Extend the splint from the elbow to the knuckles of the hand, allowing the fingers to cup over the distal edge of the splint (see Figure 15). Apply an elastic bandage to hold the splints securely in place. A fracture occurring toward the middle of the lower arm should be splinted in the same position. Apply a sling or similar support to relieve the weight of the splint and immobilize to the side of the body.

Fracture of the Elbow A fracture of the elbow is often caused by overextension of the joint. It may involve a fracture of the bones of both the upper and the lower arm. There may be extensive damage to the surrounding tissue, ligaments, nerves, and blood vessels. Do not attempt to straighten or bend the arm to splint. Immobilize or splint the arm in the position in which it was found. Figure 16*a* demonstrates an inflatable splint used to immobilize the entire arm. It also serves as a pressure

Figure 15 Applying a splint to immobilize a fracture of the forearm.

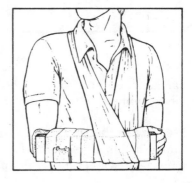

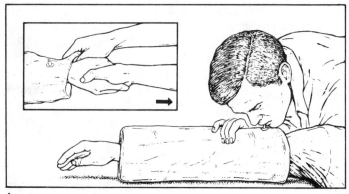

A

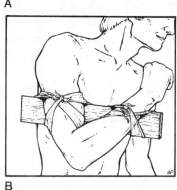

B

Figure 16 Immobilize a fracture or dislocation of the elbow in the position in which it is found. (a) Inflatable splint being applied and inflated in a straight-arm position; (b) immobilizing the elbow in a bent-arm position.

bandage over the injured elbow. Figure 16b depicts an elbow splinted in the bent-arm position.

Fracture of the Upper Arm In splinting the upper arm (humerus), pad two small pieces of wood or similar material and splint to the flat part of the arm. The splint

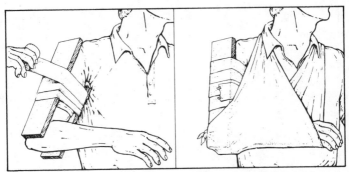

Figure 17 Immobilizing and supporting a fracture of the upper arm.

to the underside of the arm is somewhat shorter and should be well padded to protect the armpit. Secure the splint firmly to the arm prior to applying a sling for support. Strap the arm to the side of the body to immobilize (see Figure 17).

Fracture of the Foot A fracture of the foot may be caused by a severe twisting of the ankle. Most people who suffer this injury do not realize they have broken a bone in their foot. First remove the shoe and apply a small pillow splint (see Figure 18). This is an ideal method of immobilizing and protecting a fracture of the foot or the ankle. Temporary support may also be given by applying an elastic bandage and figure-eight support to the ankle (see "Sprains," Figure 1). Do not permit the victim to walk.

Note: On suspected fractures of the foot during ski accidents, it is usually best to leave the boot on until the person is brought into the aid station. It may help keep

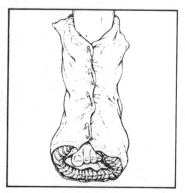

Figure 18 Using a pillow splint to immobilize a fracture of the foot.

down the swelling, and more importantly, will prevent exposure to the cold and possible frostbite. (You also account for your boot!)

Fracture of the Lower Leg (Tibia and Fibula) A fracture of the lower leg may involve both the tibia and the fibula. The tibia is the main weight-bearing bone and would be the most serious fracture of the two. In ski accidents there is often a twisting of the bone, causing a spiral-type fracture of the tibia. This type of fracture causes intense pain. In splinting this type of injury, the splint should extend at least to the knee, immobilizing the entire leg. The same basic principle should be used as in splinting the forearm. Pad well and splint along the flat part of the bone. A special technique used to splint this type of fracture is to encase the leg in a cardboard splint (see Figure 19). This splint will provide support both to the underside and to the sides of the leg. Fill the cardboard splint with packing, towels, or

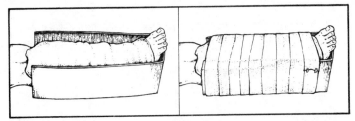

Figure 19 Using a cardboard splint to encase and immobilize a fracture of the lower leg.

similar materials. Wrap firmly with an elastic bandage. Provide a stretcher.

Fracture of the Kneecap Immobilize the kneecap (patella) using the same technique described for a dislocated knee.

Fracture of the Upper Leg A fracture of the upper leg (thighbone, or femur) is usually a very serious and painful injury. There may be a complete break, causing an override of the bones. The ideal treatment for this fracture calls for a traction splint, which involves special equipment and expertise on the part of the rescuer (see Figure 20). It is best to leave this treatment to trained medical personnel. You should immobilize the victim and splint one leg to the other. Pad the area between the legs, especially around the ankle and knee, with a blanket, towel, or similar bulky material. Use a stretcher to evacuate the victim. *Note:* If traction is used, by applying a steady pull on the leg, do not release this traction until the splint has been secured and the leg completely immobilized.

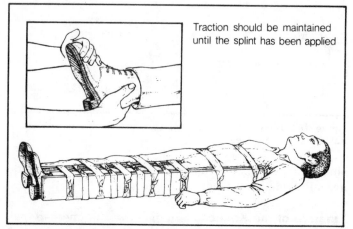

Traction should be maintained until the splint has been applied

Figure 20 Applying traction to the leg (inset) and immobilizing a fracture of the upper leg.

Fracture of the Hip Most injuries causing a fracture of the hip are due to falls or automobile accidents. There are often other injuries, especially internal injuries, associated with a fractured hip. The recommended treatment is to immobilize the injured person, treat for shock, and obtain an ambulance. (Refer to Figure 8 for position in transporting this type of injury.)

Chapter 8
Poisons and Drugs

Poisoning

Poisoning is a serious medical emergency. Poisonous substances are most likely to be ingested and include foods, drinks, drugs, and various household products. Fortunately, about 85 percent of all poisonings reported are from mildly toxic substances. In severe poisoning, if untreated, respiratory problems may develop with possible cessation of breathing. With any possible poisoning, try to determine whether poisoning actually occurred and the type and the amount of the poison that was ingested. Have the container of the substance(s) in front of you and call the hospital emergency department, the poison control center, or your physician. Follow their recommendations as to the proper antidote. If the advice of the physician or the center conflicts with the label, disregard the label; it is probably outdated. Once emergency treatment is accomplished, the victim should be referred to the hospital immediately. Bring the container of suspected poisonous substance, or any vomitus, with you to the hospital.

Poison Control Centers There are over 600 poison control centers, operating 24 hours a day, throughout the United States, where information can be obtained on suspected poisonings. The information and services of these centers are available primarily to physicians and hospitals, but also to the lay population, concerning most poisons and their best-known antidotes. The poison control center usually will have two numbers listed, one specifically for physicians and hospitals and one for the public. Keep this number near your telephone with other emergency telephone numbers. A directory of the poison control centers in the United States can be obtained from the National Clearinghouse for Poison Control Centers. Write to the U.S. Department of Health and Human Services, Food and Drug Administration, Bureau of Products Safety, 5401 Westbard Avenue, Bethesda, MD 20016.

Preventive Measures for Poisoning The best way to deal with poisoning is to prevent it from happening. A greater awareness of poison preventive principles will make any home safer. It is important to properly educate children and other family members about poisonous substances and their dangers. Safety measures around the home should include:

- Check for proper labeling, storage, and utilization of medications. Keep them secure and out of the reach of children.
- Keep all poisonous products in their original containers.
- Never provide or offer medications to other people and do not use medications after date of expiration. Use only the dosage indicated.
- Products that give off fumes should only be used in well-ventilated areas.

- Common poisonous plants should not be planted where small children are about. If in doubt, consult with nursery personnel on the various poisonous plants in your locale.

- Read safety warnings printed on the label before using any dangerous product. *Dangerous* = a taste is toxic. *Warning* = a teaspooon to an ounce is toxic. *Caution* = an ounce to a pint is toxic.

- When possible, dispose of all toxic substances down the drain or toilet, and flush out the container before discarding.

- Do not reuse bottles that have previously contained poisonous substances.

Poison's Entry into the System

Poison can enter the body by mouth, inhalation, injection, and absorption through the skin.

Poisoning by Mouth A general rule can be followed successfully for most poisonings by mouth. If the poisonous substance was intended for human consumption (to be taken into the mouth), then it should be vomited. An example of this would be contaminated food or an overdose of a medication. If the substance leaves stains and burns around the lips, throat, and mouth, it should be diluted but not vomited. If it is a petroleum distillate (gasoline, kerosene, etc.), do not treat until you call the poison center or hospital and are advised how to proceed. Inducing vomiting with syrup of ipecac is the best way to remove poison from the stomach. If a person is partly conscious, unconscious, or convulsing, do not administer fluids or induce vomiting. It is important that you provide an open airway and administer artificial respiration, if necessary.

Poisoning by Inhalation Fumes and vapors from gases or toxic substances may affect the breathing center. The victim should be removed from the area and artificial respiration administered if breathing stops.

Poisoning by Injection Poisoning caused by stings, bites, or drugs that enter the body by injection require specific treatment. Artificial respiration is necessary if breathing is affected.

Poisoning by Absorption Substances such as insecticides, cleaning fluids, acids, or other chemicals that come in direct contact with the skin should be thoroughly rinsed in water for at least 15 minutes. Refer the person to a physician or a hospital for further treatment.

Poison Control Kits Poison control kits contain two items which are considered to be the best general treatment for most types of poisoning. These kits contain syrup of ipecac and activated charcoal (see Figure 1). However, their use is advised only after consulting with a physician. Syrup of ipecac is given *only* when you want to induce vomiting. Ipecac results in vomiting within 15 to 30 minutes in most cases. It is the best method for inducing vomiting and will evacuate 30 to 50 percent of the stomach contents. *Dosage:* If the person is over 1 year of age (children to adults) give 1 tablespoon followed by 1 to 2 glasses of water. If the person is less than 1 year of age, give 2 teaspoons followed by $\frac{1}{2}$ to 1 glass of

Figure 1 Poison control kit: syrup of ipecac and activated charcoal.

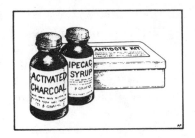

water. Most people will vomit in 15 to 20 minutes or less; however, if vomiting does not occur after 20 minutes, repeat the dosage *once only*. It is recommended that syrup of ipecac be replaced every 2 years.

Activated charcoal is effective in preventing a number of highly toxic substances from being absorbed into the bloodstream. Mix 1 to 2 tablespoons of powdered activated charcoal in an 8-ounce glass of water and drink immediately. This is usually given when you *do not* want the person to vomit. *Caution:* Do not give activated charcoal if syrup of ipecac is indicated or if a specific antidote is recommended. Activated charcoal should be used when a sizable amount of highly toxic substance which has been swallowed needs to be absorbed. This is especially the case if vomiting was induced late.

General Procedures in Poison Cases

- Estimate the amount of poison taken. Unless they have eaten pills or tablets, children under 3½ years will normally take only one bite or swallow; however, always assume they may have taken more. In children over 6 years of age, suspect a larger ingestion.

- Call poison control center, hospital, or physician.

- Induce vomiting if indicated. The use of ipecac is the single most important aspect of treatment if vomiting is indicated.

- If a small child refuses to take fluids, squeeze the cheeks to force the mouth open to get fluids into the mouth and hopefully into the stomach.

- The use of the fingers down the throat to induce gagging and vomiting is sometimes effective.

- When vomiting is induced, have the person's head and trunk lower than the hips to facilitate vomiting and prevent aspiration of the fluids.

- Flush any strong acids or alkali off the face with plenty of water.

- If breathing stops, give artificial respiration.

- Get person immediately to a hospital emergency room by car or ambulance.

- Take poison container and any vomitus with you to the hospital.

Specific Poison Treatment

- *Alkali* (corrosive): drain cleaners, oven cleaners, ammonia, electric-dishwasher detergents. Same treatment as for *acidic* products.

- *Acid* (corrosive): toilet bowl cleaners, metal cleaners, oxalic-acid products, and phenol. The treatment for both *acidic* and *alkaline* products is to administer 1 to 2 glasses of liquid, preferably water or milk. *Do not induce vomiting.* (See "Do Nots in Poison Cases," below.)

- *Petroleum distillates, gasoline, kerosene, naphtha, lighter fluids, furniture polish, and varnish removers. Do not* give treatment, call poison control center or hospital, maintain open airway.

Do Nots in Poison Cases

- *Do not* give fluid as a rule unless the person has swallowed a corrosive substance, acid or alkali.

- *Do not* induce vomiting without medical advice, especially if the poison swallowed is an acid or an alkali. It will cause additional burning of the throat and esophagus.

- *Do not* induce vomiting if the poison is a petroleum distillate.

- *Do not* neutralize alkali with fruit juice or vinegar and water. It causes a severe heat reaction, often reaching the boiling point, burning the throat, esophagus, and stomach.

- *Do not* neutralize acids with sodium bicarbonate, chalk, or soap and water. Carbon dioxide may be released, inflating and rupturing the stomach.

- *Do not* administer salt solutions, especially to small children. Repeated doses can cause salt intoxication, seizures, and death.

- *Do not* administer Epsom salts as a laxative in food poisoning. It may cause severe diarrhea and shock.

- *Do not* give a person milk to dilute camphor, phenol, or gasoline. The fat may increase the body's absorption of the poisonous substances.

Drug Poisoning

The misuse or abuse of almost any drug may cause poisoning and must be treated immediately. Listed are some general guidelines to follow:

- If it was intended to be taken by mouth, induce vomiting.
- If breathing is impaired or if the person is unconscious or convulsing, ensure an open airway.

- If breathing stops, administer artificial respiration.
- If irrational behavior is displayed, calm victim down, give reassurance, and protect from bodily harm.
- A victim who appears sleepy or drowsy should be kept awake; get the victim to stand up and walk around; apply a cold, damp towel to the victim's face and the back of the neck.
- Any serious case should be referred to a physician, hospital, or drug-abuse treatment center.

Poisonous Plants

Many plants are highly toxic when ingested in sufficient amounts and can cause severe gastrointestinal, respiratory, circulatory, and/or neurological disturbances within the body (see Table 1). Still other plants may cause severe skin irritations when contacted. Positive identification of the plants that may have been ingested or touched is essential in providing the proper treatment. Due to the high incidence of plant poisoning, individuals should become more aware of and knowledgeable about the poisonous plants in the areas where they reside or travel. Educate your children so they can identify these plants. Most victims of plant poisoning are under 5 years of age. Individuals should be aware of which part of the plant is dangerous, e.g., leaves, flowers, berries, seeds, stems, roots, or the wood. The degree of toxicity of plants varies, depending upon what part of the plant is ingested, the location in which it grows, and the season of the year it is consumed. The symptoms incurred when a poisonous plant is ingested vary with each plant.

Signs First, a burning sensation in the mouth, blurred vision, severe abdominal pains, cramps, and vomiting or diarrhea. (The signs may develop in as little as 20 minutes or may take several hours before becoming apparent.) Second, a rapid heart beat, sweating, nausea, muscular weakness, and confusion may be present. (Some plants cause mental confusion, depression, hallucinations, stupor, and comalike conditions.) In severe cases an individual may go into convulsions or shock and have cardiac or respiratory problems.

Treatment Keep the victim's airway open. If the person is conscious, dilute the poison and induce vomiting. Give fluids by mouth and treat for shock. Provide artificial respiration if necessary and take the victim immediately to the hospital.

Plants That Pose Special Problems A number of plants pose special problems if a piece is placed in the mouth. The plants in question often cause severe swelling of the throat, resulting in dificult swallowing, breathing, and speaking. The air passage may become entirely closed, causing an acute respiratory emergency. Dumb cane is one of the worst offenders. Other common plants in this category include caladiums, chinaberry, elephant's ears, and philodendrons (see Figure 2).

Specific Plants That Irritate Plants that cause severe skin irritations through the secretion of their oils should be avoided. Contrary to common belief, complete immunity does not exist, and highly susceptible individuals may suffer severe reactions upon exposure. Irritations

TABLE 1
Common Poisonous Plants Found throughout North America

Below is a list of plants that may be injurious to a person's health and if taken in sufficient quantity may result in death. Noted is the part of the plant that is considered most toxic and the primary bodily function that is affected.

Plant	Part	Plant	Part	Plant	Part
Aconite[a]	G,R	Bushman's poison[a]	G,N,R	English ivies[a]	N,I
American wild plums[a,i,j]	G	Caladiums[a]	G,N	English laurel[b,i]	N
Apples/cherries[b,i]	G	Carolina jesamine[a]	R	False hellebores[a]	G,R
Angel's-trumpet[a]	N	Castor bean[a]	G,N	Fava, or Horsebean[h]	G
Apricots/peaches[b,i]	G	Chinaberry[b,g,i]	G,N	Four-o'clock[a]	G
Autumn crocus[a]	G,C	Crown of thorns[a]	—	Foxglove (Digitalis)[a]	C,G
Azaleas[a]	N,C	Daffodil[c]	G	Glory lily[a]	G,R
Baneberry[a]	G,C	Daphnes[a]	G,R	Hollies[b]	G
Belladonna[a]	C	Death camas[a]	G,C	Horse chestnuts[a,h,i]	G,N
Bird-of-paradise[c,h]	G,I	Delphiniums[a]	N,G	Hyacinths[c]	G
Black locust[d,i,j]	G,N	Dumb canes[a]	N,R	Hydrangea[a]	G
Bleeding hearts[a]	G	Elderberries (varieties)[a,k,i]	G	Inkberry[a]	G,I
Boxwoods[i]	G	Elephant's ears[a]	G,N,R	Iris[a]	G
				Jack-in-the-pulpit[a]	G

134

Plant	Systems
Jerusalem cherry[a]	G,C
Jimsonweed[a]	G,N
Jonquil[c]	G
Lantanas[d,m]	C
Larkspur[a]	I,N
Lily of the valley[a]	G,C
Locoweed[a]	N
Locust (black/white)[d,h,l]	G
Mandrake[j,l,m,n]	G,R
Marijuana (hemp)[a]	N
Mayapple[j,l,m,n]	G,R
Mescal bean[h]	G,N
Milkbush[a]	I
Mistletoe[b]	G,C
Monkshood[a]	G,R
Morning glory[h]	N,G
Mushrooms (poison)[a]	G
Naked lady[c]	R
Narcissus[c]	R
Nightshades (most)[a]	G,R
Nutmegs[h]	N,R
Oaks (acorn)[a]	G
Oleander[a]	G,N
Opium poppy[l,m]	N
Peyote[a]	G,N
Philodendrons[a]	N
Poinsettia[a]	I
Poison hemlock[a]	R,N
Poison oak, ivy, sumac[a]	I
Pokeweed[a]	G
Potatoes[b,l,i,n]	G,C,R
Privets[b,l]	G,N
Rattlebox[h]	G,C
Rhododendrons[a]	G,C
Rhubarb[l]	G,R
Rosary pea (love bean)[b]	G,C
Sky-flowers[b]	R
Sweet peas[h]	N
Thorn apple[a]	G,N
Virginia creeper[b]	G
Water hemlock[a]	G,N
Wild/Indian tobaccos[a]	G,C
Wisteria[h]	G
Yaupon[b]	G
Yellow jessamine[a]	G,C
Yew[h,s,l]	G,R

Notes: C = circulation, G = gastrointestinal, R = respiration, N = neurological, I = irritation, [a] = entire plant, [b] = berries, [c] = bulb, [d] = bark, [e] = bud, [f] = fruit, [g] = flowers, [h] = seeds, [i] = shoots, [j] = stems, [k] = wood, [l] = leaves, [m] = unripe berries/fruit, [n] = roots/rootstocks

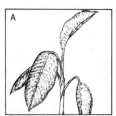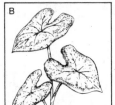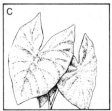

Figure 2 Plants that present special problems if placed in the mouth or eaten: (a) dumb cane, (b) caladium, (c) elephant's ear.

can result from direct contact, the handling of exposed pets, or even through smoke inhalation during the burning of poison oak. Specific plants that cause irritation include the arnica, buttercup, crowfoot, four-o'clock, iris, mayapple, oleander, poinsettia, primrose, stinging nettle, and yew. The stinging and/or itching occurs immediately after contact with the plant.

Treatment The treatment consists of thoroughly washing with a strong soap-and-water solution, rinsing off the affected area several times. Application of a mild antiseptic or lotion is often helpful in relieving itching. Severe cases should be referred to a physician. *Note:* Irritation from the stinging nettle may be lessened by applying an insect repellent containing at least 70% *N,N*-diethyl-*meta*-toluamide.

Poison Ivy, Poison Oak, and Poison Sumac These are perhaps the most prominent plants that cause severe skin irritations. The recognition and avoidance of these plants are important preventive measures (see Figure 3). If

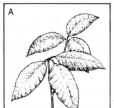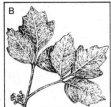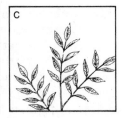

Figure 3 Plants that may cause severe irritation if touched or contacted: (*a*) poison ivy, (*b*) poison oak, (*c*) poison sumac.

contact is suspected, affected areas should be thoroughly washed. Use special care to keep your hands away from your face, especially the eyes and mouth. Clothes should be removed and laundered in hot water and strong soap. Pets who contact poison oak, ivy, or sumac must also be bathed, as they can carry the resin for several days.

Signs Normally symptoms will not develop for several days after contact. When present, there is a reddening of the skin, a rashlike appearance, and a burning and itching sensation. Blisters will form and seep or ooze a watery substance. In severe cases, considerable edema and swelling will be present.

Treatment Numerous anti-inflammatory commercial preparations for application to the lesions are available. The gels and liquids, i.e., Topsyn Gel, Rhuligel, and Derma Pax, appear to be superior. Creams cause "crusting over" of the blisters and do not dry up the sore as quickly. It is important to keep the areas clean and avoid scratching between applications to prevent secondary infection. Scratching will not spread the dermatitis once the person has bathed with soap and water. For larger areas, cool saltwater (2 teaspoons per quart) compresses are helpful in relieving itching. Apply for 10 minutes four times daily. Individuals with severe problems should consult with their physician.

Chapter 9
Things That Bite and Sting

There are thousands of venomous insects, animals, and forms of marine life which one might encounter every day of the year and which pose a potential threat to our safety. Most of these creatures, however, are far more wary of humans than we are of them. They usually employ their poisonous toxin against people only as a mechanism of self-defense. Fortunately, most of these creatures inhabit areas far from our shores. For the ones that do reside in the United States, antivenins are available to counteract most severe cases of envenomation when treated properly.

Bees, Wasps, Yellow Jackets, and Hornets

It is estimated that nearly 1 percent of the population is insect allergic, and half of that 1 percent possess a high sensitivity to the sting. *Most sensitive individuals are unaware of the seriousness of their problem.* Stings from these insects account for many more deaths per year than do snakebites (Figure 1). These deaths are not usually

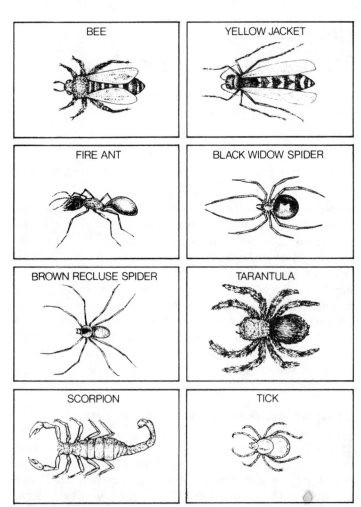

Figure 1 Common venomous insects found throughout North America.

caused by the envenomation itself but to an anaphylactic shock reaction that creates respiratory problems because of swelling of the vocal cords and constriction of the bronchial tubes. It is a potentially life-threatening condition. Sensitive individuals should consult with their physician, who may consider a desensitization technique with the use of whole-body or whole-venom antigens. These persons should obtain a special antivenin emergency kit for beestings. Preventive measures are encouraged, especially after rains and during the seasons when these insects are most noticeable. Since bees are especially attracted to bright colors, floral prints, lotions, strong perfumes, and scented soaps, use of these should be avoided. Other safeguards against stings from these insects range from the wearing of shoes in the outdoors to the covering of foods at picnics. The wasp, hornet, and yellow jacket may sting repeatedly, injecting venom with each thrust of their tail. Bees normally leave their stinger with its venomous sac in the victim's skin. Immediately remove the sac, as it can release venom for an additional 15 to 20 minutes.

Signs The sting produces a fierce burning sensation followed by reddening and itching at the site. Swelling, pain, and a large, firm white welt will soon appear. Advanced signs in the sensitive person include headache, nausea, weakness, anxiety, abdominal pains, chest constriction, and difficulty in breathing. This may be followed by the classic signs of shock and unconsciousness.

Treatment Take special care not to squeeze the venomous sac. Flick out by using a pointed object such as a nail file. Apply an ice bag or cold compress to all stings for at least 15 minutes. A paste made from meat tenderizer and water is effective in neutralizing the toxin. Sensitive individuals should be immediately given the antivenom injection (Ana-Kit), treated for shock, and referred to a hospital.

Ants, Chiggers, Fleas, Mites

Ants both bite and sting. The bite or sting of the fire ant, found primarily in the South and Southeastern United States, is very severe, perhaps the most toxic of all ant bites. When encountering this insect, a person is often bitten or stung many times. The greatest danger is to the highly sensitive person and to infants. The nonsensitive person will usually survive with no ill effects. Anaphylaxis kits (requiring a prescription) are available. Mites, chiggers, fleas, bedbugs, and lice that come in contact with the body can become very irritating and should be removed.

Signs The symptoms of the bites from the fire ant are similar to the hornet sting. Other bites from many insects will leave small welts, possibly some blistering, and cause considerable itching.

Treatment The treatment for the fire ant bite is to apply an ice bag or a cold compress to the area for at least 15 minutes. For other insect stings and bites, take a hot bath, lathering off several times with a strong soap and rinsing thoroughly. Apply an antiseptic solution to the welts. Be sure to thoroughly launder clothes and bedding.

Spider Bites

Spiders account for only a few deaths annually, and these occur primarily among children. The most common poisonous spiders in the United States are the *black widow* and the *brown recluse,* or *violin spider.* The bites of two South American stowaways, the South American tarantula and the banana spider, are extremely venomous, but fortunately rare in the United States. The venom from these spiders is more potent than that of most venomous snakes, but a considerably smaller amount is injected. The spider is considered a "loner" and nonaggressive, with the exception of the brown recluse and the South American tarantula. When spiders bite, they usually cling, making them easy to retrieve and identify. Most spider bites occur in attics, cellars, outdoor latrines, woodpiles, and abandoned buildings. Care should be taken when entering any of these areas. Individuals bitten by poisonous spiders should be referred to a physician for possible hospitalization.

Black Widow The female black widow is three to five times larger than the male and is not considered aggressive. She has a glossy black body and variations of a red or yellowish orange hourglass marking on her abdomen. The male has a smaller marking of the same color on his abdomen, resembling a small dot. The male, due to his small fangs, has more difficulty than the female in penetrating the skin, but his venom is equally toxic.

Signs The appearance of a small pinprick is often followed by a dull, numbing pain developing between 15 and 60 minutes. This pain spreads gradually to other parts of the body, causing tightness and cramping of the muscle around the bite. Little, if any, swelling results until 1 to 2 hours after the bite, and too often the bite is neglected. The victim's abdomen may become boardlike, with excruciating pain and spasms. Headache, eyelid swelling, extreme restlessness, anxiety, vomiting, muscular weakness, and sweating develop. A skin rash may develop with an increase in skin temperature.

Treatment Thoroughly cleanse the wound with soap and water. An ice cube or ice bag may relieve pain. Treat for shock and refer the person to a physician or hospital as soon as possible. The spider should be taken also. BCLS should be provided if necessary. Individuals under age 16 and over age 65 or with hypertension should be hospitalized. An antivenin has been developed, but is rarely needed for those between the ages of 16 and 65, unless the person has unusually severe symptoms or is pregnant.

Brown Recluse (Violin Spider) There are at least 10 species of this spider, all of them venomous. They are about 1 inch in length when the legs are fully extended. They can be identified by the violin-shaped marking on their backs. They are masters of the "hit-and-run" tactic and are often difficult to catch.

Signs Usually a mild stinging sensation occurs after the bite. Later a small hard spot develops at the site with a reddening around a small blanched area. The bitten area may become red, swollen, and tender during the initial 10 hours. *A red ring encircles the bite* (reminiscent of a bull's-eye on a target). Further signs and symptoms include skin rash, chills, hives, nausea, and vomiting.

Treatment   The treatment is essentially the same as for the black widow bite. Early identification and referral to a hospital is important. Treat any secondary infection as normal wound management. There is no antidote for this spider at the present time.

Other Spiders   The *Phidippus* is a crablike jumping spider that somewhat resembles the black widow. It is smaller and black in color, with red or orange markings on the abdominal dorsum. The *Filistata* is a smaller spider with heavier legs that is often mistaken for the brown recluse. Tarantulas commonly found in the United States are nonaggressive, and their bite is quite mild. The bites of the jumping spiders and trapdoor spiders may produce a mild local reaction. All spiders are considered venomous, but fortunately their small fangs cannot often pierce the skin. The greatest danger of any of these spider bites is to small children, and when a child is bitten, it is very important that the spider be captured and identified.

Signs   A slight burning sensation is often present with signs resembling a small pinprick from the bite. This is followed by itching, swelling, and redness at the site. The swelling and amount of edema present varies with the type of spider that inflicts the bite.

Treatment   Wash the bite thoroughly with soap and water. Place an ice cube or cold pack on the area to relieve swelling and reduce the pain. Aspirin or anti-histamine is recommended if available. Especially treat children against shock.

Scorpions Most North American scorpions are relatively harmless and do not sting unless provoked. They can cause considerable pain, however, when they do sting. The venom is injected by the stinger in the scorpion's tail. Children are most vulnerable and may require an antivenin. The scorpion located in the Southwest (Arizona, New Mexico, and Lower California) is small in size, and its venom is very potent.

Signs The sting causes immediate and severe pain, numbness, and a tingling sensation of the part affected. The injured part becomes sensitive to touch or movement. General muscular weakness may occur with the possible paralysis of the extremity involved. Other signs include nausea, muscle contraction, gastric distension, and, in extreme cases, convulsions and respiratory problems.

Treatment Immediate cold compress or ice bag should be applied to relieve the pain. Ammonia solution also may relieve pain when applied to the site. A specific antivenin is called for with the Southwestern scorpions, especially with children. Further treatment may include BCLS and/or a quick trip to a hospital. Experts recommend that children be hospitalized.

Tick Bites Ticks are present in almost all wilderness and wooded areas and are most prevalent during the late spring and early summer. They are small, hard, flat, oval-shaped creatures about $\frac{1}{8}$ to $\frac{1}{4}$ inch in length. Certain species carry serious diseases such as Rocky Mountain spotted fever (tick fever, tick typhus) and Colorado tick fever. Preventive measures should be taken in infested areas by keeping well-clothed and buttoned up, spraying liberally with a good insect repellent containing 70% or more Deet (*N,N*-diethyl-*meta*-toluamide), and inspecting one another after the day's hike. Ticks usually attach to the skin where it is thin with protective hair growth, e.g., the armpits, head, groin, and buttocks. Animals become infested easily.

Signs Infection brings chills, fever, headaches, and muscle aches, and the victim experiences a general overall aching condition. A red rash may appear on the limbs. This condition may go away and recur several days later.

Treatment To remove the tick, swab it with alcohol, gasoline, or kerosene, which may cause it to release and back out. A burnt match, cigarette, or ember can also make them release. In removing the tick with tweezers, work it out gently and slowly to avoid crushing the insect and so that all parts of its head are removed. Do not crush the tick. Drop it into the fire. The bite should be scrubbed carefully with soap and water and an antiseptic solution applied. If the bite becomes inflamed and swollen or if the victim develops a fever, a physician should be consulted.

Venomous Worms, Mosquitos, and Flies

Leaches Leaches are small, bloodsucking, wormlike creatures often inhabiting stagnant lakes and ponds. They will attach themselves to any part of a person swimming or wading.

Treatment   Placing a burnt match, lighted cigarette, ember, or hot paperclip on them will force disengagement. A pinch of salt may also be used to kill them. Wash the wound thoroughly with soap and water and apply an antiseptic solution.

Mosquitos and Flies   These insects are always irritating and some can inflict very painful and sometimes infectious bites. Black flies, deer flies, horseflies, and many varieties of mosquitos are present in most wilderness areas, especially around lakes and streams. The best prevention is to use an insect repellent containing 70% or more Deet (*N,N*-diethyl-*meta*-toluamide). Keep all parts of the body covered and obtain a good mosquito netting for the head while hiking and sleeping.

Treatment   For bites, scrub the part thoroughly with a strong soap and water, and apply an antiseptic solution liberally to the welt. A cold compress may give some relief.

Snakebites

The most common poisonous snakes in North America are the *rattlesnake,* the *copperhead,* the *cottonmouth water moccasin,* and the *coral snake* (see Figure 2). The first three are pit vipers and have the common characteristics of a hinged pair of long fangs, vertically slit pupils, a flat head wider than the neck, and a pit (sensing organ) between the eye and nose. All species of rattlesnakes account for nearly 60 percent of all snakebites and almost all snakebite-related deaths. Fatalities are not common,

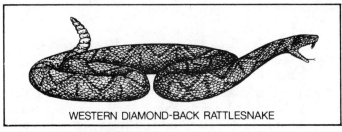

WESTERN DIAMOND-BACK RATTLESNAKE

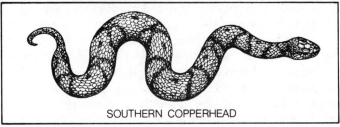

SOUTHERN COPPERHEAD

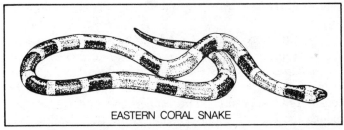

EASTERN CORAL SNAKE

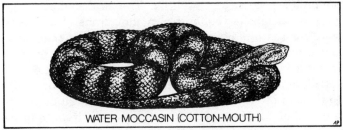

WATER MOCCASIN (COTTON-MOUTH)

Figure 2 Common poisonous snakes found in the United States.

averaging only 12 to 15 per year. However, children, elderly people, and individuals with hypertension are the most vulnerable. Most reported snakebites occur on the hands, arms, and legs. Staying on the trails, using a stick to beat the ground, placing your hands carefully while climbing (especially in crevices and holes), and maintaining alertness around streams and areas of poor visibility, are all sound preventive measures in snake country.

Snakes are most noticeable between 9 a.m. and 9 p.m. but most active between 3 and 6 p.m. They prefer temperatures between 60 and 90°F, and cannot tolerate temperatures over 110°F. They are considered fairly inactive, but may strike, in temperatures below 40°F. In approximately 20 percent of all snakebites no venom has been injected, and in many cases only a small amount is injected.

Of the more than 32 rattlesnake species identified, the most lethal are the *eastern diamondback,* the *Mojave,* the *red diamond,* and the *western diamondback.* However, it must be recognized that all species should be considered dangerous. The copperhead and the cottonmouth moccasin are not considered life threatening, but can produce edema and swelling. The coral snake seldom bites, although its venom is very dangerous. The treatment for the bite of a coral snake is different than that for the pit vipers. Specific antivenins have been developed for most snakes, but they are not normally recommended outside of the hospital. It is estimated that approximately 80 percent of all bites reported occur within 20 minutes' travel time to a hospital. A most essential item to have with you in case of snakebite is the keys to your car. Of even greater importance is to have the car for a quick trip to the hospital!

Signs Poisonous snakes (pit vipers) will leave one, two, or sometimes three fang marks, often hindering the recognition of the bite. Nonpoisonous snakebites leave several rows of teeth marks, making them fairly easy to distinguish (see Figure 3). If venom has been injected, it often produces instant burning and swelling around the fang marks and edema within the first 5 minutes. There may be a tingling sensation of the tongue in as little as 20 seconds after the bite, with a subsequent numbness extending to the mouth, scalp, and fingers that increases in severity within a few moments. The tingling of the tongue is often associated with a rubbery or metallic taste. A bluish discoloration at the general site of the injury may occur 8 to 12 hours after the bite. The victim

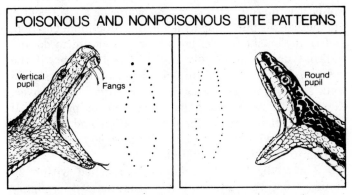

Figure 3 Comparison of the poisonous (pit viper) and the non-poisonous snakebite.

is often nauseated and may lose consciousness. If there is no swelling after the first $\frac{1}{2}$ hour and there are no apparent symptoms, it is still important to observe the bite for at least 4 hours and treat it as a puncture wound. *Caution: systemic signs may be delayed* with the mojave, speckled, panamint, and several other rattle-snakes.

Note: There are 32 species of rattlesnakes and over 65 subspecies found in North, Central, and South America. Fifteen of these species are found in the United States.

Treatment If a medical facility is within 20 minutes' travel time, use the following procedure: get the victim away from the snake because it may strike again. Keep the victim lying down; quiet and reassure him or her. Place a constricting band 2 to 3 inches above the bite or joint (i.e., on the side closer to the trunk). Cleanse the wound thoroughly with soap and water or an antiseptic; immobilize the part at heart level, in a functional position, and treat for shock. Do not allow the victim to do any walking unless absolutely necessary. However, if the victim needs to walk from the scene, he or she should walk slowly and rest every 3 to 5 minutes. Avoid over-exertion but get to the hospital as soon as possible. If possible, kill the snake for identification and take it to the hospital with the victim. Call ahead so that a proper antivenin can be made available.

If a medical facility cannot be reached within 20 minutes, use the same initial procedures of thoroughly cleansing the wound and application of the constriction band. Make lengthwise cuts $\frac{1}{8}$ inch deep and $\frac{3}{8}$ inch wide through each fang mark with a sterile blade within 5 minutes after the bite. Use the suction cup provided in snakebite kits for at least 30 minutes to 1 hour (see Figure 4). Use of mouth suction is acceptable if no other method is available. The venom poses no danger to the rescuer if sores are not present on the mouth and the rescuer spits out the blood and venom. If the cuts are made within 3 minutes, it is estimated that 10 to 12 percent of the injected venom can be removed. Normally, little venom can be removed after 30 minutes. However, in the case of children, an extra 30 minutes may be enough to save a life. Complete the first aid by treating the wound and the victim for shock. Take the person and the dead snake to a hospital immediately. *Do not* give any alcoholic beverages to the victim. A tetanus booster is usually recommended.

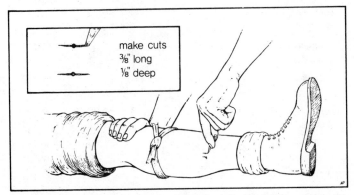

Figure 4 Treating a poisonous snakebite (pit viper) if travel time to a medical facility is over 20 minutes.

Antivenin is recommended only in a hospital setting because the victim needs to be tested initially for sensitivity to horse serum. A minimum of three vials of antivenin is the initial effective dosage, and in severe cases five to eight vials are recommended. Children require larger doses of antivenin, often twice that of an adult. Antivenin should not be given if it is suspected that the snakebite did not release any venom.

TABLE 1
Poisonous Snakes of the World*

Poisonous Snake	Length, in	Venom, mg
North America		
Rattlesnakes:		
Eastern diamondback	32–65	200–850
Western diamondback	30–65	175–600
Red diamond	32–52	120–450
Timber	32–54	75–210
Prairie	32–46	35–110
Southern Pacific	32–48	75–250
Great Basin	32–46	75–150
Mojave	22–40	75–150
Sidewinder	18–30	18–58
Pigmy rattlesnake	24–30	12–35
Massasauga	24–38	15–45
Cottonmouth	30–50	90–145
Copperhead	24–36	40–70
Eastern coral	16–28	2–6
Western coral	15–18	1–6

* Indicates the average length and the approximate yield of dry venom of a number of dangerous snakes. The amount of venom does not reflect the toxicity of the poison.

Rattlesnakes The eastern diamondback may reach 6 feet or more in length. It may inject a considerable amount of venom; twice as much as its western counterpart, or the red diamond (see Table 1). Its poison is considered to be about three times as deadly. The mojave bite causes little edema and swelling and is often mistaken for minimal envenomation. It is considered to be much more lethal than the western diamondback and accounts

TABLE 1
Poisonous Snakes of the World (Continued)

Poisonous Snake	Length, in	Venom, mg
Central and South America		
Tropical rattlesnake	20–48	20–40
Barba amarilla pit viper	46–80	70–160
Bushmaster	70–110	280–450
Europe		
European viper	18–24	6–18
Africa		
Puff adder	30–48	130–200
Saw-scaled viper	16–22	20–35
Green mamba	50–72	60–95
Asia		
Indian cobra	45–65	170–325
Common krait	36–48	8–20
Russell's viper	40–50	130–250
Malayan pit viper	25–35	40–60
Australia		
Tiger snake	30–56	30–70
Indo-Pacific		
Beaked sea snake	30–48	7–20

Source: Adapted from Finlay E. Russell, M.D., *Snake Venom Poisoning,* Lippincott, Philadelphia, 1980, p. 154.

for most of the snakebite deaths in California. The recommended treatment is to double the amount of antivenin that would ordinarily be administered. The Great Basin, Southern Pacific, prairie, timber, sidewinder, and other species are all considered less dangerous than the red diamond.

Cottonmouth This snake is normally found around the water in the Southern United States and is more aggressive than the rattlesnake. It may reach 3 to 4 feet in length. Its venom produces considerable swelling and ecchymosis (discoloration), and an antivenin is necessary in the treatment of the bite.

Copperhead Copperheads are rarely over 3 feet in length and their bite produces a considerable amount of swelling and edema. The greatest concern is secondary infection resulting from the bite. However, in severe envenomation of a small child or elderly person an antivenin is recommended for treatment.

Coral Snake The coral snake averages less than 2 feet in length, is very shy, and seldom bites. The eastern coral is quite lethal, and experts recommend a specific antidote to be given at once. The western coral snake is not considered nearly as dangerous.

The snout of the coral snake is always black and has bright black, yellow, and red rings encircling the body. The yellow rings always separate the black and red rings. It is often mistaken for the scarlet snake but can easily be remembered by this saying: "Red on yellow will kill a fellow. Red on black, venom it will lack."

The coral snake has several pairs of short, fixed fangs at the front of the upper jaw, and, because of its short size, uses a chewing motion to inject the venom. Most bites occur on or between the fingers. It is estimated that 50 percent of all the eastern coral bites are fatal if untreated.

Signs The fang marks are very difficult to see and may appear as tiny scratches. The signs of envenomation take time to develop, and often deterioration proceeds so rapidly that an antidote may not be successful unless given immediately. Only minimal signs of pain and swelling are usually present.

Treatment Immediately wash the area thoroughly with soap and water or an antiseptic. Keep the victim quiet and give reassurance. Normally do not apply a constricting band or make any incisions. However, if the victim is more than 1 hour from a hospital, a constricting band may be placed just above the bite area. It should be released every 10 minutes until medical help is obtained. If possible, call ahead to the hospital so that an antivenin may be made available. Do not give any beverages or foods. Bring in the dead snake for identification. Persons suspected of having been bitten by a coral snake need 48-hour hospital observation.

Nonpoisonous Snakes The nonpoisonous snakebite is identified by the rows of teeth marks inflicted during the bite. The teeth make a number of tiny sharp puncture wounds. Swelling and edema may occur around the wound.

Treatment   First get the victim away from the snake. Wash the wound thoroughly with soap and water. Treat the wound as a puncture wound. Apply mild disinfectant and a dry, sterile dressing. Refer the victim to a physician for further evaluation and a possible tetanus shot.

A poison control center for snakebite is located in Oklahoma City, Oklahoma, and provides a publication called the *Antivenin Index*. It lists all the known venomous snakes and other important venomous animals, the required antidotes, and the nearest supply outlets. The cost of this index is $3.00.[1]

Poisonous Marine Life

The most common venomous species of underwater marine life found in American waters include the stingray, jellyfish, sea urchin, scorpion fish, and catfish (see Figure 5). Most venomous creatures inhabit the warmer coastal waters of the South Pacific, Australia, and other parts of the world. People residing in the areas of southern California, Florida, the Caribbean, and the Gulf of Mexico should be aware of the poisonous marine life in their areas. Injuries from marine life in these waters may be very painful but are not usually fatal. Complications can occur, so follow-up treatment is strongly advised. Most of the injuries are obtained while wading, swimming, or fishing. Standard treatment for these venomous stings

[1] Poison Information Center, Oklahoma Children's Memorial Hospital, P.O. Box 26307, Oklahoma City, OK 73126; telephone (405) 271-5454.

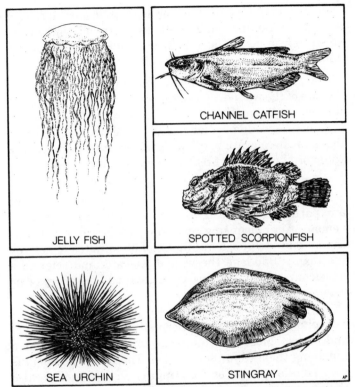

Figure 5 Common venomous marine life found in American waters.

is now well established. Children are especially vulnerable and must be given special attention for any sting.

Stingray The stingray (whipray) has a long, whiplike tail equipped with arrowlike barbs. If it is stepped on it lashes out with its barbed tail, inflicting a penetrating wound, usually to the foot or leg. It leaves a ragged wound, contaminating it with the torn integumentary sheath or spines. The venom may affect the cardiovascular, respiratory, or nervous system.

Signs A sharp, intense, throbbing pain occurs at the site of the wound. The pain is very severe and reaches its greatest intensity in less than 90 minutes. A laceration or puncture wound is made, often bleeding freely. Swelling and discoloration of the part occurs. Parts of the spine or sheath may break off and stay in the wound.

Treatment Immediately and thoroughly irrigate the wound with cold *salt* water to remove the venom. Remove any parts of the sheath, as they will continue to release venom. After cleansing, soak the part in water as hot as can be tolerated for a minimum of 30 minutes to destroy the toxin. Bandage the wound, elevate, and refer to a physician. Treat for shock. A tetanus booster may be recommended.

Scorpion Fish This fish is normally found in deep waters and rocks. Most injuries occur to divers or fishermen removing them from their hooks. The scorpion venom is very similar to that of the stingray. The stonefish, also of this family, is not found in American waters.

Signs A small, incisive puncture wound with throbbing pain, increasing in intensity, occurs. The pain will radiate to the groin or axillary area. The wound may become swollen and cyanotic. Signs of shock, possible loss of consciousness, and respiratory or circulatory collapse may occur in severe cases.

Treatment The sting is more difficult to irrigate than that of the stingray. The use of a syringe to rinse the wound thoroughly with salt water is recommended. The use of hot-water follow-up treatment recommended for the stringray is also advised. Provide BCLS if necessary. A specific antivenin is available.

Jellyfish (Portuguese Man-of-War) The jellyfish stings are inflicted by their long tentacles and range from mild irritation to excruciating pain. Most of the stings occur on the legs, and the greatest danger is that the victim may go into anaphylactic shock and drown.

Signs The pain may vary from a mild pricking sensation to violent burning. The pain may remain localized or radiate up the extremities, with pain and cramps developing in the muscles and joints. Redness, swelling, and a rash appear. Other symptoms may include pallor, weakness, anxiety, chills, nausea, and vomiting. Signs of shock, respiratory problems, and paralysis of the part may develop in only a few minutes in severe cases.

Treatment Immediately pour salt water over the injured part, irrigating thoroughly. Attempt to remove all the tentacles, wearing gloves while removing. Pour 95% alcohol over the wound. The use of rubbing alcohol, ammonia, or vinegar is acceptable if 95% alcohol is not available. Next, apply meat tenderizer to neutralize the toxin. Dust off the area with talc, flour, a dry powder, or dry sand, and scrape off the stingers with a dull blade. Once again, rinse the area with salt water. Obtain medical assistance.

Fire and Stinging Corals These sea creatures inflict pain with their tentacles somewhat like the jellyfish, but the wounds are not nearly as severe. The anemones and hydras are of this family.

Signs See "Jellyfish," above.

Treatment Immediately cleanse the area thoroughly with a soft brush or coarse cloth and soapy water. Rinse off with alcohol and then with a hydrogen peroxide solution. Apply a sterile dressing to prevent infection and refer to a physician. Serious cases call for rest.

Catfish The catfish often inflicts a laceration-type wound. The venom it releases produces an instant stinging and throbbing pain at the site. Later the pain may radiate up the affected limb. The area may become swollen, red, and cyanotic. In untreated cases numbness, edema, and gangrene may appear around the wound.

Treatment Cleanse and irrigate the wound thoroughly; apply hot water as in the treatment for the stringray. If prompt treatment is rendered, this wound is not likely to be a problem. However, lack of treatment may cause a serious secondary infection.

Other Marine Life

Moray Eel, Turtles, and Sharks Cleanse the wounds thoroughly, control any bleeding, bandage, and treat for shock. Obtain medical assistance.

Sea Urchins, Cone Shells, and Spiny Fish Treat by irrigating thoroughly in salt water and inactivating the toxin in hot water; remove any spines and treat similarly to stingray.

Octopus Syringe the wound of the octopus bite with a strong soap solution. Obtain immediate medical attention. BCLS may be necessary.

Puffer Fish, Scromboids, and Shellfish These fish poison through ingestion. Proper identification is very important. If they are eaten, respiratory or circulatory collapse may occur. Give the victim BCLS and refer immediately to a hospital. Activated charcoal may be of some value if given early enough. Antihistamines are also helpful in shellfish poisoning.

Chapter 10
Burns

Burns are classified according to degree—*first, second, third,* and *fourth*—identifying the depth of tissue destruction. This depth is often difficult to determine due to the variance in the thickness of the skin and the fact that burns will frequently be of mixed depths. Burns are most commonly caused by heat and radiation, but they are also caused by chemicals, electric current, and the cold. Injury from burns results in various degrees of skin and tissue destruction. The amount of body surface and the depth of the burn are important in determining the seriousness of the injury. The method of determining the extent or amount of the body surface that is burned is referred to as the *rule of nine* (see Figure 1).

Thermal Burns

The most common burns are those due to heat and are referred to as *thermal burns*. The problems associated with severe burns are pain, infection, fluid loss, and shock. These problems become increasingly serious ac-

Figure 1 The *rule of nine* used to estimate the approximate area of body surface injured or burned.

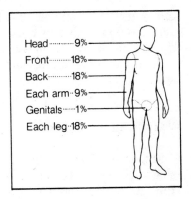

Head ⋯⋯⋯ 9%
Front ⋯⋯⋯ 18%
Back ⋯⋯⋯ 18%
Each arm ⋯ 9%
Genitals ⋯⋯ 1%
Each leg ⋯ 18%

cording to the degree and the amount of body surface damaged. Burns are more serious for the very young, the elderly, and individuals in poor physical condition. The prompt treatment of a serious burn can reduce the amount of pain and decrease the element of shock. Infection is not usually a problem with first- and second-degree burns, as the inner layers of the skin have not been exposed.

Treatment The general rule for treatment of first- and second-degree burns if less than 20 percent of the body surface is burned (15 percent in children) is ice-water therapy followed by application of a dry, sterile dressing if blisters develop. Soak the dressing in ice water and apply to the wound. The purpose of the ice water is to relieve pain and discomfort, reduce the swelling, and possibly retard blistering. In more serious burns (third- and fourth-degree), where the inner layers of the skin have been exposed, there is serious danger of infection and scarring. Apply a dry, sterile dressing, treat for shock, and immediately obtain medical assistance. *Note:* The use of cold water does not apply to large burns, as it can cause a hypothermic condition (see "Hypothermia" in Chapter 11).

Classification of Burns

First-Degree Burns First-degree burns involve superficial tissue damage affecting the outer layer of the skin. Sunburns, contact with hot objects, and mild scalds are examples.

Signs There is a general redness of the skin and some pain and discomfort.

Treatment Immerse the part in cold water; apply an ice bag or a cool, wet cloth over the area for 10 to 20 minutes. If pain is severe or persists, apply mild sunburn cream and give aspirin. *Note:* Some sunburn preparations contain the "caine"-type drugs which sensitize the skin and cause rashes. Perhaps it is best for some people to avoid over-the-counter preparations for sunburn.

Second-Degree Burns Second-degree burns involve the first two layers of the skin and may vary in depth. Severe sunburns, flash burns, and burns caused by hot grease or scalding are examples.

Signs Injury causes pain and blister formation with moistness and redness of the skin.

Treatment Treat the same as for first-degree burns,

with cold-water therapy. For small burn areas, cold compresses may be applied for 1 to 2 hours to relieve the pain. Carefully dry the areas after the cold-water therapy and apply a dry, sterile dressing over any blisters. Grease burns should be cleansed by patting the area with a sterile gauze soaked in a mild soap-and-water solution. Sunburn creams are not recommended for second-degree burns. Give aspirin to relieve pain, treat for shock, and refer to a physician.

Third-Degree Burns Third-degree burns involve the deeper layers of the skin, with damage to the nerves, blood vessels, sweat glands, and some muscle damage. These burns may be caused by flames, ignited clothing, chemicals, electricity, or immersion in hot water. Infection and shock are two primary considerations.

Signs The skin is white and charred, and the possibility of complete loss of the outer layer of skin exists. If this is the case, there will be a complete lack of sensation to touch.

Treatment Apply a dry, sterile dressing or freshly ironed sheet as quickly as possible. Do not remove any clothing adhering to the burn, but *cut away* surrounding material if necessary. Treat for shock and immediately obtain an ambulance. (For guidance in applying a dressing to a burn, refer to Figure 16 in Chapter 6, "Dressing and Bandaging Wounds.")

Fourth-Degree Burns Fourth-degree burns are more extensive and are called *char burns*. They extend into the subcutaneous tissue, underlying muscle, and possibly the supporting bone. These burns may be caused by intense heat, electricity, nuclear radiation, or molten metal.

Signs The skin is completely charred with loss of all layers of the skin.

Treatment The treatment is the same as for third-degree burns. *Note:* Serious burns cause severe pain and considerable loss of body fluids from the tissue. If untreated, moderate to severe shock may occur.

General Considerations for Burn Treatment

- Do not open blisters, as this increases the possibility of infection.
- If blisters break, special wound care should be taken to prevent infection.
- Do not remove any clothing adhering to the burned area.
- Remove all rings, watches, and bracelets, as severe swelling is likely to occur.
- Keep person warm with a sheet, blanket, or coat to aid in preventing shock.
- Do not use any salves, ointments, or antiseptics on burns of second degree or more.
- Elevate hands, arms, or feet if they are burned.
- Second-degree burns of 15 to 30 percent of the body surface are considered serious, and the victim should be evacuated from wilderness or remote settings.
- Third-degree burns of more than 2 percent of the body surface are considered serious.

- Any burns on the face and neck are dangerous, due to the possibility that inhaled fumes may create respiratory problems.
- Any burns in the mouth and nose are dangerous and may cause respiratory problems.
- Any deep second- or third-degree burn in the young or aged is considered serious.
- Any electrical burns are serious and may need BCLS.
- Burn victims at high altitude should be given oxygen if possible.

Chemical Burns

Chemical burns are common in schools, industry, and laboratory areas.

Treatment   All chemical burns should be thoroughly flushed with lots of water. Use a shower or running water. All clothing involved should be removed during the shower and discarded. Seek medical attention.

Burns of the Eyes   These burns are usually caused by chemicals that are splashed into the eyes.

Treatment   Flush the eyes for at least 5 minutes for an *acid* and 15 to 20 minutes for an *alkali*. Allow a gentle flow of water from a faucet to run over the eyes (see Figure 2). *Caution: Use only water.* After flushing, cover the eyes with a dry, sterile dressing and refer to the hospital. If medical care is unavailable, flush alkali burns for a longer time—hours if necessary.

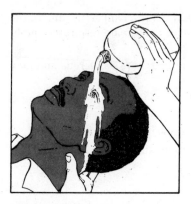

Figure 2 Rinse the eye with copious amount of cool, running water.

Electric Burns

Electrical burns may result from direct contact with electric power or lightning. The greatest concern with any electrical burn is respiratory or circulatory failure. A secondary consideration is the possibility of considerable tissue destruction in the accompanying wound.

Treatment   Provide BCLS if necessary and obtain an ambulance. Care must be exercised in removing any person from an electric current by disengaging the power or removing the wire with a nonconducting material. Treat the wound with a dry, sterile dressing, and treat the victim for shock.

Burns from Cold

Burns from the cold are caused by the skin coming in direct contact with extremely cold metal. Direct contact of the skin with any metal object in a cold situation is an example.

Treatment   Disengage the skin from the metal by flushing with warm water. If water is unavailable in the outdoors, urinating on the part stuck may be the last resort in releasing it. Apply dry, sterile dressing. *Caution:* If the temperature is very cold, do not use cold water to flush as that may make it worse. Gently teasing the skin off the metal is safer.

Chapter 11

Abnormal Temperatures: Heat and Cold

Few of us like to be very hot or very cold, but sometimes exposure to extreme temperatures is more than simply a matter of comfort. Sometimes it involves a serious medical problem.

Heat Problems

Prolonged exposure to an extremely hot, humid environment may lead to heat cramps, heat exhaustion, or heatstroke. Most heat problems can be prevented with proper adjustment to the environment and an adequate fluid and salt intake. It is estimated that up to 2 quarts of fluids can be lost in an hour through perspiration during hot and humid conditions. Needless to say, if this fluid loss is not replaced, varying degrees of dehydration will result.

The best method of avoiding serious fluid loss and heat disorder is to follow these sound preventive measures:

- Wear light-colored, loose-fitting clothing which will reflect the sun's rays.

- Keep as much of the body protected from the sun as possible and wear a light-colored, wide-brimmed hat.

- Rest in the shade during the hottest part of the day and minimize activity.

- Drink lots of fluids and add salt liberally to your food. Eat cool foods and drink extra fluids, even if not thirsty.

- Avoid sudden changes in temperature (e.g., going in and out of air-conditioned places); cool off the interior of an automobile by opening the windows prior to entering.

- Limit your exposure to the sun, especially when moving up in altitude. In a hot environment, allow 15 minutes of exposure the first day and increase 15 to 30 minutes daily for the first 7 to 10 days.

- Avoid strenuous outdoor activity during hot periods, especially if the temperature is over 85°F and the humidity is over 60 percent.

- When exercising or working in hot temperatures, take frequent rests and replace fluid and salt loss.

- Do not use plastic or nylon sweat clothing to lose weight as they reduce the evaporation of the perspiration from the skin, preventing appropriate heat loss.

- Individuals on a low-salt or salt-free diet should take special precautions in activity or exercise during hot periods.

- If you feel tired and nauseated or have headaches, dizziness, or muscle cramps, stop any activity, get plenty of rest, and drink lots of fluids. Seek medical assistance if the condition persists.

Heat Cramps Heat cramps or muscle cramps are spasmodic, painful contractions of the muscles which may last up to 15 minutes or longer. A person who is most likely to experience these cramps is someone in good physical condition who has overexerted during hot, humid conditions. The tightening or cramping condition of the muscle is usually due to a salt and/or fluid loss or imbalance which needs to be corrected.

Signs Profuse sweating, severe muscle cramps, and pain, especially in muscles of the legs or the abdomen. Faintness, dizziness, and exhaustion may be present.

Treatment Remove the victim to a shady location or cool room and give a salty liquid (1 teaspoon of salt to a quart of water, lemonade, Gatorade thirst quencher, etc.). Rest and inactivity are important. Gently stretch the leg muscles by pulling the toes up to relieve the pain. The person should rest for at least 12 hours prior to resuming any additional activity. *Do not massage the muscle or give salt tablets.*

Heat Exhaustion Heat exhaustion is usually caused by extreme physical exertion and excessive sweating over a prolonged period of time in a hot environment. Alcoholic beverages, dehydration, excessive vomiting, or diarrhea all increase a person's susceptibility to heat exhaustion. This condition resembles a mild form of shock.

Signs The person is listless, fatigued, and faint. Skin is ashen, cool, and damp, and the person is often sweating profusely. Weakness, dizziness, headache, nausea, blurred vision, irritability, and mild muscular cramps are common. Temperature is normal and pulse is thready and elevated, possibly to 100 beats per minute. In severe cases the victim is in a semiconscious or unconscious condition (see Figure 1).

Treatment Loosen clothing; place the person in a reclining position in a cool environment. Administer cool water or a saltwater solution by mouth. Cool the person down by removing the clothing and sponging with cool cloths or rubbing alcohol. Stop all of the victim's activity and institute rest for at least 24 hours. Normally this condition is easily reversed and nonfatal; however, if the person does not respond well to treatment or appears overly fatigued, refer immediately to a hospital. These individuals should rest 2 to 3 days, drink lots of fluid, and salt their food liberally.

Heatstroke A heatstroke (sunstroke) is one of the least common but most serious of the heat problems. It is a profound disturbance of the heat-regulatory mechanisms of the body, associated with the cessation of sweating. A

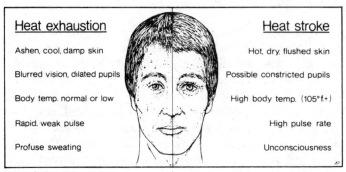

Figure 1 A comparison of the signs and symptoms of heat exhaustion and heatstroke.

person who experiences a heatstroke has been in a hot, humid environment (such as occurs in a heat wave) over a prolonged period of time. It can be likened to the thermostat breaking on a car. If the temperature is not controlled, the brain will literally cook. Individuals who have a high incidence of heatstroke include the elderly, those with respiratory and/or circulatory problems, alcoholics, and those who have difficulty acclimating to various temperature changes. When sweating ceases, the heat builds up within the body with the temperature rising to 105°F or higher. This temperature must be immediately reduced or death may occur.

Signs The onset of heatstroke is rapid. Initially, the person experiences headache, nausea, and weakness. Later, signs of confusion, lack of coordination, and lapse into unconsciousness may occur. Skin is hot, flushed, and dry, and the person appears feverish. Pulse rate is high, up to 160, and temperature is elevated to 105 to 110°F (see Figure 1).

Treatment The victim's temperature must be immediately reduced below 100°F. Immerse in a cool tub of ice water, use an alcohol rub, or cover with wet sheets and/or blankets soaked in cold water. Vigorous massaging with cold cloths or ice cubes is valuable in reducing the temperature. When temperature is reduced, keep the victim in a cool, well-ventilated place. Immediately obtain an ambulance and medical assistance. *Caution:* Prolonged cold after temperature has been reduced may cause hypothermia.

Heat Asthenia Heat asthenia is a heat-related problem associated with people under conditions of stress, often in a hot environment.

Signs Headache, giddiness, fatigue, body inefficiency and weakness, lack or loss of strength, debility, insomnia, and loss of appetite. Precordial pain, high pulse rate, and palpitations upon exertion may be present.

Treatment Removal from stressful situation, and hot environment. Provide rest and have victim drink plenty of fluid with a salt solution. Refer to a physician.

Prickly Heat Prickly heat is an irritating skin rash common to activity and physical exertion in hot weather. The sweat glands become impaired and do not function properly.

Signs Skin becomes red and inflamed. Itching and an irritating rash occur.

Treatment Get away from the heat; bathe in cool water three or four times daily, drying thoroughly and changing clothes frequently. Attempt to reduce or avoid sweating by staying in a cool environment. Avoid using creams or ointments, as they clog the pores and inhibit proper function.

Injuries Caused by Cold

Extreme cold, as well as heat, can cause problems for the unprepared or unprotected.

Frostnip and Frostbite Frostbite injuries may be superficial or deep, depending upon the degree of exposure to the cold and the extent of the tissue damage. Injuries of this type are common to the face, ears, hands, and feet where the exposure is the greatest and the circulation the poorest. Several factors lead to these conditions: cold, dampness (including perspiration), wind, lack of body heat production, and fatigue or exhaustion. Any exposure to a damp, cold condition may result in frostnip. As this condition persists, various degrees of frostbite will occur and the tissue may die. The continued exposure to the cold and dampness combined with wind and lack of heat production may lead to a more serious problem called *hypothermia*. In this condition, which is life-threatening, the temperature of the inner core of the body drops considerably.

Frostbite can occur at any altitude. However, the higher the elevation the greater the incidence. This risk factor increases with a fall in air temperature combined with the wind, making the effect of the cold more severe. Any wound in which the tissue is already damaged is extremely susceptible to frostbite.

The best way to prevent these injuries is to have the proper dry clothing, keep out of the wind, and maintain adequate nutrition. Proper clothing is discussed in the outdoor section of the guide. Smoking and alcohol should be avoided in a cold environment. Smoking will constrict the blood vessels of the skin, making the tissue more susceptible to frostbite. Alcohol dilates the blood vessels near the surface of the skin, increasing the loss of body heat.

Frostnip   Frostnip is caused by a cold condition and is often referred to as first-degree frostbite. This injury is usually to the face, earlobes, nose tip, fingers, or toes. The injury is similar to that of a mild to a severe sunburn. If promptly recognized and treated, it is generally not a problem.

Signs   Initial redness, swelling, and a tingling and painful sensation of the affected part. The frozen area becomes numb and waxy, leaving a firm, white cold spot at the site.

Treatment   The best treatment is rapid rewarming. This can be accomplished with the use of unaffected hands or a warm object, placing the hands under the armpits or on the abdomen. Exercise by wiggling the toes, gently clapping the hands, or jumping. (Do not rub the hands *vigorously* together, as this may damage tissue.) Put on dry wool socks or mittens if the hands or feet are wet. Drink hot beverages such as soups, broths, or warm cider. Getting out of the cold environment is most important as the injury may develop into a more severe case of frostbite.

Frostbite   Frostbite is classified in degrees ranging from first to fourth. The longer you are exposed to the cold, wind, and dampness, the greater the frostbite injury becomes. You can usually tell if a part of the body is frostbitten by the feeling of numbness or a "clublike" sensation. Frostbite may be painful initially, as in frostnip, but as the condition becomes more severe, sensation of the part is lost. Most frostbite occurs at a temperature between 30 and 50°F with a prevailing wind. For example, a calm-air temperature of 40°F with a 20-mph wind equals an effective air temperature of 18°F (see Table 1).

Signs Frostnip conditions exist initially, and as the freezing continues, sensation of the part is lost. Numbness, swelling, edema, and blisters develop. As freezing continues, skin becomes waxy; dead white, blue, or black; and solid on pressure.

Treatment Get out of the cold. Severe frostbite cases should be evacuated and hospitalized as soon as possible. If medical help is not available, thaw the part by immersing it in warm water 100 to 105°F (to touch of normal skin) for 20 to 40 minutes. *Thawing should be done only if medical help is not available and there is no chance of refreezing.* A deep reddening of the skin will develop with considerable pain during the rewarming process. After rewarming, very gently dry the part with a warm towel; apply loose, sterile gauze dressings; and cover with a warm blanket. Give the person lots of hot fluids: soups, broths, hot cider, tea, etc. The person must be kept warm and treated for shock, and the injured parts should be elevated. Prevent infection with meticulous cleanliness. The follow-up treatment includes daily warm soaks (100°F) for 15 minutes (boil the water initially and add a germicidal soap while cleansing). Place sterile gauze wedges between the toes or fingers and wrap the affected area loosely with a sterile gauze. Maintain warmth with blankets or towels wrapped around the injury and elevate the injured part. A tetanus booster is indicated. *Caution:* Once the frostbitten part has been thawed out, do not go back out into the cold. If you must

TABLE 1
The Wind-Chill Factor[*]

Wind Speed, mph	Temperature (Thermometer Reading, Degrees Fahrenheit) Equivalent Temperature at Indicated Wind Speed																		
	50	40	35	30	25	20	15	10	5	0	−5	−10	−15	−20	−25	−30	−35	−40	−50
Calm	50	40	35	30	25	20	15	10	5	0	−5	−10	−15	−20	−25	−30	−35	−40	−50
5	48	37	33	27	21	16	12	6	1	−5	−11	−15	−20	−26	−31	−36	−41	−47	−57
10	40	28	21	16	9	4	−2	−9	−15	−24	−27	−33	−38	−46	−52	−58	−64	−70	−83
15	36	22	16	9	1	−5	−11	−18	−25	−32	−40	−45	−51	−58	−65	−72	−77	−85	−99
20	32	18	12	4	−4	−10	−17	−25	−32	−39	−46	−53	−60	−67	−75	−82	−89	−96	−110
25	30	16	7	0	−7	−15	−22	−29	−37	−44	−52	−59	−67	−74	−83	−88	−96	−104	−118
30	28	13	5	−2	−11	−18	−26	−33	−41	−48	−56	−63	−70	−79	−87	−94	−101	−109	−125
35	27	11	3	−4	−13	−20	−27	−35	−43	−51	−60	−67	−72	−82	−90	−98	−105	−113	−129
40	26	10	1	−6	−15	−21	−29	−37	−45	−53	−62	−69	−76	−85	−94	−100	−107	−115	−132
	Cold Condition			Very Cold Condition			Bitter-Cold Condition												
	Little danger if properly clothed			Greater danger			Very dangerous condition, even if properly clothed												

[*] The wind-chill factor has a dramatic effect on cold temperature. For example, if the temperature reads zero (0°F) and there is a 25 mph wind, the equivalent temperature or chilling intensity equals a −44°F on a calm day. Wind speeds greater than 40 mph have little additional effect on temperature.

Note: Dampness (being wet) combined with cold increases a hypothermic condition even to a greater degree.

Source: Adapted and reproduced from *Patient Care*, Patient Care Publications, Darien, Conn. Copyright 1977. Used by permission.

continue in the cold, *do not* thaw. Individuals who have sustained frostbitten parts are more susceptible to subsequent cold conditions. Specific recommendations on frostbite include:

- *Do not* immerse the frozen part in cold water.
- *Do not* rub the frozen parts with snow or anything cold.
- *Do not* massage or rub the injury, as it may destroy more tissue.
- *Do not* apply any salves or ointments to the injury.
- *Do not* rewarm by placing in an oven or in front of an open fire.
- *Do not* walk on the frozen toes after thawing.
- *Do not* go back out into the cold. Avoid the *freeze-thaw-freeze* sequence which is more hazardous than leaving the part frozen.

Other Injuries due to Cold and Damp   Cold injuries can be sustained at temperatures above freezing as a result of prolonged exposure to a cold, damp environment. These injuries—chilblains, immersion, or trenchfoot—usually affect the hands and feet.

Signs
Chilblains   Affected part is red, swollen, hot, and tender to touch, and there is frequently itching of toes and fingers.
Immersion Foot   Cold, numb, swollen feet; a pale, waxy, clammy condition.

Treatment   Dry and warm the part carefully. Apply warm, moist towels followed by the donning of warm, dry wool socks or mittens. Rest and drink hot liquids. If blisters appear in immersion foot, take measures to prevent infection.

Hypothermia   Hypothermia is a cooling of the body-core temperature to a level where the normal muscular, mental, respiratory, and circulatory activity is affected. It is usually caused by exposure to a low or rapidly dropping temperature, compounded by dampness and wind. This condition can, and often does, occur at temperatures well above freezing, especially if there is a high wind-chill factor present. The wind-chill factor is an important reference in determining an accurate, effective temperature value and the possibility of cold injuries. Visual estimation of the wind velocity can be made as indicated in Table 2.

Hypothermia is one of the leading causes of death in the wilderness where cold, damp conditions suddenly develop. Inexperienced or ill-prepared people have difficulty sustaining themselves under these adverse weather conditions. A wet, cold, windy environment brings a rapid loss of body heat which can cause a hypothermic state. Special precautionary measures must be taken to guard against any heat loss in a cold environment.

Body heat is lost by the mechanisms described below and as illustrated in Figure 2.

Radiation   Direct heat is transferred from the body by the discharge or emission of energy. The conservation of heat can be aided by wearing a hat and gloves. Body heat can be gained by radiation from the sun, a fire, food, and exercise. Follow this rule: If your feet are cold, cover

TABLE 2
Visual Estimation of Wind Velocity

Wind Speed, mph	Observed Phenomena	Descriptive Terms
0–1	Smoke rises vertically; flag lies limp	Calm
1–3	Smoke drift shows direction of wind; leaves on trees move slightly; flag barely moves	Light air
4–7	Wind is felt on face; leaves rustle; flag occasionally moves out a little from staff	Light breeze
8–12	Leaves and small twigs are in constant motion; flag stands out from staff at 30–45° angle	Gentle breeze
13–18	Dust is raised; loose paper blows about; small branches move	Moderate breeze
19–24	Small trees begin to sway; flag stands out at 90° angle	Fresh breeze
25–31	Large branches are in motion; whistling is heard in telephone wires; flag stands out straight from staff and flutters vigorously	Strong breeze

32–38	Whole trees are in motion; it is inconvenient to walk against the wind; light, loose objects are lifted from the ground; flag whips about wildly	Moderate gale
39–46	Twigs are broken off trees; automobile in motion trembles; telephones lines whine loudly	Fresh gale
47–54	Trees bend sharply; slight structural damage may occur; both vehicles and pedestrians are seriously impeded	Strong gale
55–63	Trees may be uprooted; structural damage is considerable	Whole gale
64–72	Severe damage occurs	Storm
72+	Walking against wind is nearly impossible; destruction is widespread	Hurricane

Source: Reprinted from: George L. Cantzlaar, *Your Guide to Weather*, Barnes & Noble, New York, 1964. Used by permission.

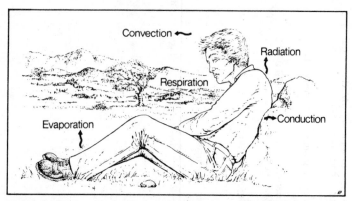

Figure 2 Body heat loss occurs rapidly in a cold, damp, and windy environment, especially if the individual is poorly clothed.

your head. This will aid in preventing loss of body heat through radiation.

Evaporation (Sweating)   Heat is lost by perspiration or sweat from the skin being evaporated into the air. This heat loss is increased through exercise. Several layers of clothing allow ventilation, and the water vapor passes through without saturating the clothing.

Respiration (Air Expelled from the Lungs)   Body heat is lost through respiration. Cold inhaled air is warmed by exposure to blood flowing through the respiratory passages and lungs (to body temperature). When this air (now warm) is exhaled, heat is lost from the body. In extremely cold weather, if you breathe through a wool scarf it will reduce body heat lost through respiration.

Conduction   The heat is transferred directly away from the body when in contact with a cold surface, such as snow, cold ground, or water. For example, if you sit on a block of ice, you will lose heat directly to the cold object. Rain-soaked or sweat-saturated clothing removes body heat at an exceedingly high rate. Wearing dry clothing and insulating the body from a cold surface are important in preventing this heat loss.

Convection (Wind)   The body is continuously warming a layer of air next to the skin to nearly body temperature. If this layer of warm air is constantly removed by the wind or by cold-water immersion, there will be a rapid increase in body heat loss. The body temperature is regulated by the clothing we wear, with the dead air spaces between layers of clothing preventing rapid heat loss.

The failure to wear a hat and gloves at an air temperature of 40°F may account for nearly half of the loss of total body heat. The body heat loss, especially from wet skin caused by excessive sweating, immersion, or rain, is greatly increased by the wind and cold (see Figure 2). Clothing saturated with water loses up to 90 percent of its insulation properties against the wind and cold conditions. Physical exertion increases the evaporation of body fluids and depletes the body's supply of energy by burning up calories. Awareness of the causes of hypothermia is perhaps the most important aspect of its prevention. Basic measures include:

- Avoid dampness caused by perspiration, immersion, or rain.
- Wear warm, dry clothing, using the layer method (see "Clothing and Equipment" in Chapter 18).

- Carry the proper rain and wind gear, emergency plastic shelters such as tents, ground cloth, or lawn cleanup bag.
- If dampness occurs, replace wet clothing with dry, warm clothing.
- Avoid tight clothing, especially gloves and shoes, to maintain adequate circulation.
- Maintain at least minimal activity to generate body energy.
- Limit activity that causes excessive perspiration; avoid undue fatigue and exhaustion.
- Provide shelter to avoid the wind, cold, and/or rain (make camp early in storm conditions).
- On wilderness trips, not shaving or washing the face gives protection from the cold.
- Provide nutrition to supply body needs (eat small snacks often, especially high-energy foods, e.g., hard candy, salted nuts, dried fruit, or trail mix).
- Avoid use of tobacco and alcohol at low temperatures.
- Provide adequate water intake, hot fluids, and fruit juices if available.
- Be alert to the early signs and symptoms of hypothermia by using the buddy system.
- Rewarm individuals who are shivering or showing early signs of hypothermia.

The early recognition of the signs of hypothermia is essential in preventing this problem from becoming a serious medical emergency. The simple tasks of striking a match or buttoning and zippering clothing are often difficult to manage during the onset of hypothermia. If any of these signs develop, activity should stop and every effort be made to get the person into a warm, dry environment.

Signs Goose pimples, shivering, undue fatigue, stumbling, forgetfulness, and mental confusion are early signs of hypothermia. These symptoms are associated with low body-core temperature and are an indication of progressive body heat loss. As the body temperature continues to be reduced, progressive muscular, mental, and circulatory problems appear, at the approximate temperature levels indicated in the list below. To determine body temperature, obtain a special thermometer with readings below 95°F, e.g., a Kodak multipurpose developing thermometer.

98 to 95°F Sensation of chilliness, goose pimples, inability to perform minor tasks with the hands.

95 to 93°F Increased muscle incoordination; slow, labored movements; stumbling pace; violent shivering; and mild confusion.

93 to 90°F Extreme muscle incoordination, frequent falling and stumbling, difficulty in speaking, inability to use hands, and signs of depression.

90 to 86°F Shivering stops, severe muscle incoordination, inability to walk, confusion, irrational behavior, thinking unclear, sleepiness.

86 to 82°F Muscles become rigid, semiconscious condition, stupor, loss of contact with reality, pulse and respiration slowed.

82 to 78°F Unconsciousness, heart beat and respiration erratic.

Below 78°F Respiratory and cardiac failure and probable death. Death may occur before the body reaches this temperature level, if the heart goes into ventricular fibrillation.

The basic principles of emergency medical care for hypothermia are the prevention of any further heat loss, rewarming of the person as quickly as possible, and recognition of any complications, especially respiratory or circulatory failure.

Treatment The person must be warmed and reassured. Move the person out of the wind and cold, replacing wet clothing with dry, warm clothing. Apply external heat by building campfires, preheating sleeping bags, or providing body heat from another person. The placing of a second person in a sleeping bag to provide warmth (body-to-body contact) is one of the most effective methods of rewarming an individual in the wilderness. The use of hot-water bottles or warm stones wrapped in towels will help preheat the sleeping bag. If the person is conscious, give hot fluids, soup, tea, candy, dried fruits, etc. Add sugar or glucose tablets to fluids for quick energy. If the person's temperature drops below 82°F, artificial respiration and CPR may be necessary. This person needs to be evacuated and provided with immediate medical care. Oxygen should be administered if available. Immersion in a tub of warm water 105 to 110°F is another effective method of rewarming. If the clothing is frozen, immerse the person fully clothed, as clothes are difficult to remove when frozen. Continue to add warm water to regulate the water temperature because the cold, wet clothes cause further drop in temperature. Remove the clothing as practicable. Dry the person thoroughly and place in a warm bed until normal temperature returns. *Note:* Individuals will start to shiver violently as they emerge from hypothermia.

Severely exposed individuals have been revived when their core temperature has dropped to as low as 70°F and no visible signs of life (detectable respiration or heartbeat) were present. In one case, cardiopulmonary resuscitation was administered for over 4 hours and the person was removed by helicopter to the hospital. The blood was rewarmed through a heat exchanger and a heart-lung machine, bringing the temperature back to normal. This indicates that sustained efforts should be made to rescue individuals who have been exposed to the severe conditions of a cold environment.

Chapter 12
Medical Emergencies

Certain medical emergencies must be recognized and given special attention. Not only is it important to identify the problem, but in many instances obtaining prompt medical assistance may save a life. Specific steps outlined in the examination of the body for injuries will assist in determining the type and extent of the medical problem and the appropriate response (refer to Chapter 2, "Examination of Injuries").

Unconsciousness

There are numerous causes of unconsciousness, ranging from simple fainting to serious illness. Unconsciousness may be very brief or may last a long time. The cause of the condition is not always obvious, and determining it requires an orderly and systematic approach. In treating unconsciousness, first, and most importantly, ensure an open airway. Check the vital signs of breathing, pulse, pupil size, skin color, etc. Ask observers what happened. Check for a Medic Alert or similar tag. Based on the information from this examination, carry out the appropriate treatment. Seek immediate medical assistance.

Heart Disorders

A heart attack is one of the most common and serious medical emergencies. According to the American Heart Association nearly 650,000 persons will die of a heart attack each year, 350,000 before reaching the hospital. Many of these deaths will occur shortly after the onset of the symptoms. The average victim waits 3 hours before seeking help. If individuals obtained medical assistance within 4 minutes after the first signs occurred, most would survive. It is important to recognize the *early warning signs* of a heart attack (see Figure 1).

Early Warning Signs of Heart Attacks

- Prolonged, oppressive pain or unusual discomfort occurs in the center of the chest, behind the breastbone.
- The pain may radiate to the shoulder, arm, neck, or jaw, usually on the left side. (Sharp, stabbing pains are usually not signals of a heart attack.)
- The pain and discomfort is often accompanied by sweating, nausea, vomiting, and shortness of breath.
- Sometimes these signs subside and then return.
- The pain experienced is likened to a giant steel band being tightened around the chest, someone squeezing the heart with the fist, or an extremely heavy object or weight being placed upon the chest.

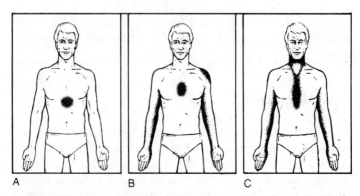

Figure 1 Early warning signals of a heart attack. Pain in one form or another usually accompanies a heart attack. The pain may vary from a mild ache to severe. (a) Pain in upper abdomen, often mistaken for indigestion; (b) pain in center chest area, inside arms, more often on left side; (c) pain in neck area, jaw, ear-to-ear, inside arms, chest. Any number of these symptoms may be present.

- If the early warning signs last 2 minutes or more, seek immediate medical assistance. Application of rhythmical coughing is advisable every 1 to 3 seconds until medical assistance is obtained (see "The Cough as a CPR Technique" in Chapter 4).

Risk Factors of Heart Disease   It is generally believed that the control of the risk factors associated with heart disease may significantly reduce heart attacks. The American Heart Association identifies the leading risks associated with heart diseases as:

- *Elevated cholesterol*   An individual with a cholesterol count of 250 or more stands three times the risk of heart attack and stroke as an individual with a cholesterol level below 194.

- *Cigarette smoking* An individual who smokes more than one pack a day runs nearly twice the risk of a heart attack as a nonsmoker.
- *High blood pressure* A person with a systolic pressure over 150 runs more than twice the risk of a heart attack and nearly four times the risk of a stroke as a person with systolic pressure under 120. (Also see Glossary, *hypertension*.)

The combination of these three risk factors may increase the incidence of heart attack up to 10 times. Males are more prone to heart attack than females. Other less well accepted risk factors subject to change include:

- Elevated triglycerides
- Lack of regular exercise
- Stress
- Obesity
- High-salt diet
- Heredity

Medical authorities believe that the reduction of the risk factors can lessen the risk of a heart attack. Any person having several of these risk factors should obtain a medical examination.

Types of Heart Disorders

Heart attacks are often referred to as *angina* (angina pectoris) or a *coronary* (acute coronary thrombosis or myocardial infarction). When a heart attack occurs, blood flow to a portion of heart muscle becomes inadequate. A portion of the heart muscle is affected and will die. The remainder of the heart muscle usually continues to contract to various degrees, depending upon the amount of heart muscle that is damaged. If the blood supply is insufficient or totally blocked to a significant area of the heart, the person may not survive. CPR can assist in maintaining oxygenated blood to the brain until the individual is transferred to a hospital where, hopefully, recovery will be possible.

Angina   Angina is a pain syndrome experienced by individuals who suffer from diminished blood supply to the heart. It is associated with a serious heart problem. Angina is caused by a narrowing of the coronary arteries that supply the heart with blood. It may be aggravated or precipitated by stress, excitement, overactivity, heavy exertion, or heavy eating. Often individuals who have completed a heavy meal pass their attack off as an acute case of indigestion.

Signs   There is discomfort or difficulty in breathing, and pains and tightness in the chest. Pain may radiate to the neck, jaw, or left arm. It may disappear after a few moments of rest (also see "Early Warning Signs of Heart Attacks," above).

Treatment   Place the victim in a comfortable semi-recumbent position to make breathing easy (prop up the back with a couple of pillows). If medication is required, help the patient to take it; e.g., place the medication under the tongue. Consult immediately with the victim's physician.

Coronary The pain associated with a coronary thrombosis resembles angina, but it is usually more intense and prolonged. A blood clot forms, causing blockage of the coronary artery, thereby decreasing the oxygen supply to the heart muscle. This is a serious medical emergency and may lead to death.

Signs Severe chest pains radiate to the neck, jaw, and left arm; the victim experiences difficulty in breathing, anxiety, weakness, sweating, pallor, cyanosis, and cold skin, especially in the extremities. Pulse may be weak, rapid, or irregular (see "Early Warning Signs of Heart Attacks," above). *Note:* Sometimes the only sign present is chest pain.

Treatment The person should be placed in a comfortable semirecumbent position. If the victim is on medication, give assistance in taking it. Obtain an ambulance or helicopter to evacuate the victim to the hospital. Give oxygen if available. If pulse cannot be felt and there are no signs of breathing, provide CPR.

Cardiac Dyspnea Cardiac dyspnea is a heart condition manifested by undue shortness of breath. It is often associated with heavy exertion, especially at high altitudes.

Signs The signs are rapid pulse rate and respiration; anxiety, sometimes with appearances of suffocation; difficulty in getting one's breath; and labored breathing.

Treatment Complete rest; give oxygen if available and evacuate to a hospital. A physician may advise a diuretic.

Other Medical Conditions

Some chest pains are not associated with heart disease. Recognition of these common chest pains is important to both the physical and mental well-being of the individual. They may result from extreme anxiety or fear or from a nervous condition. They are often associated with trembling, dizziness, and difficulty in breathing. Chest pains may also be caused by unaccustomed physical work or exercise involving the large muscles of the chest, e.g., heavy lifting, toting heavy packs, or cross-country skiing.

When chest pains occur, stop activity, and get some rest. Seek medical advice.

Heartburn   Heartburn is referred to as *acid stomach* and often occurs after a heavy meal or after drinking strong coffee, tea, or an alcoholic beverage. It often occurs when the person is lying down.

Signs   Heartburn is a burning sensation that rises up from the chest and possibly into the throat and neck.

Treatment   Rest; take milk or an antacid such as Maalox or Mylanta. Avoid foods and beverages that may cause this condition. If it is a regular occurrence, consult a physician.

Pleurisy   Pleurisy is an inflammation of the pleura, the membrane that covers the lungs and lines the inner wall of the chest cavity. Pleurisy is often associated with other diseases such as pneumonia. It is extremely uncomfortable, especially at high altitudes.

Signs   The onset of the symptoms is usually very sudden, with sharp and stabbing pains in the chest wall during respiration. Any movement or deep breathing aggravates and increases the pain.

Treatment Give aspirin and a mild sedative and refer to a physician.

Stroke (Apoplexy) A stroke is caused by the clogging or bursting of a blood vessel in the brain. Strokes cause nearly 200,000 deaths and afflict approximately 2 million people annually. They generally occur in people over the age of 40 and are associated with high blood pressure and arteriosclerosis (hardening of the arteries).

Signs The onset of a stroke is usually very sudden. The initial signs may include weakness of the arms or legs with tingling pains and numbness. Blurred vision or partial blindness and difficulty in speaking may be present. Breathing may be irregular and noisy, the face flushed, and the pupils unequal. The person may lose consciousness and/or suffer paralysis of the face, arm, or leg.

Treatment Most important is to ensure an open airway and obtain medical help by ambulance. Make the person as comfortable as possible, with the head and chest slightly elevated. Loosen clothing around the neck and waist. Treat for shock. Be prepared to handle any vomiting or convulsions that may occur. Give BCLS if necessary.

Asthma Asthma is usually caused by an allergic reaction to pollen, dust, foods, etc. It is referred to as *wheezing breathing* and affects the respiratory system. Individuals who have asthma need more time to become acclimated to higher altitudes, and often experience breathing difficulties when over 8000 feet above sea level. They should be under the care of a physician and should obtain the necessary medication prior to any wilderness outing.

Signs There is difficulty in breathing, especially during expiration. Coughing and wheezing are present. Nasal congestion may be present, and often the person will cough up large amounts of mucus.

Treatment Essentially, give supportive measures during the attack. Try to keep the person calm and quiet. Give an increase of fluids along with the prescribed medication. If the person has an inhaler or bronchodilator, help the victim to use it. Steam inhalation is often of value.

Diabetes Diabetes is a disease in which the body is unable to manage its food intake adequately. The body is unable to utilize its intake of carbohydrates and fats due to the individual's lack of insulin. The careful regulation of insulin is important for diabetics.

Diabetic Coma A diabetic coma occurs when the body does not get enough insulin to fully metabolize the carbohydrates and fats.

Signs The face is dry and flushed. Other signs and symptoms include air hunger (deep respiration), acetone breath (the smell of nail polish remover), dry skin, intense thirst, weak and rapid pulse, nausea, and vomiting.

Treatment This person needs insulin and medical attention. Administer large amounts of fluid by mouth if the person is conscious (1 teaspoon of salt per quart of water).

Insulin Shock (Hypoglycemia) Insulin shock is a condition in which the body has too much insulin. This may be caused by insufficient food intake or too much insulin.

Signs There are severe shock conditions: ashen-white color and moist, cold, clammy skin. Respirations are normal or shallow with strong and rapid pulse and perhaps unconsciousness.

Treatment Obtain immediate medical attention. Victim needs sugar. Give sugar and water (2 to 3 teaspoons per glass) or orange juice if the person is conscious. Treat for shock.

Appendicitis Diagnosing appendicitis is often difficult. The pain usually occurs initially in the pit of the stomach and gradually moves to the lower right quadrant (the lower right quadrant is the abdominal area between the right thigh and the belly button). The person may have *rebound tenderness,* in which the pain increases when you release your hands from the abdominal wall. If the appendix bursts, the pain may disappear. It will return in several hours with a sharp increase in body temperature. *Note:* The exact location of the appendix will vary in different people, and the pain will not always be located on the lower right side.

Signs Signs are tiredness, loss of appetite, nausea and vomiting, and pain in the pit of the stomach that later moves to the lower right side. Rebound tenderness may be present. Fever may be present up to 100 to 102°F.

Treatment *Give nothing by mouth.* Victim should rest in a comfortable semisitting position. Apply cold compress to the lower right quadrant. Obtain medical help. *Do not* give any laxatives.

Chapter 13

Diseases, Infectious Disorders, and Common Medical Problems

A number of illnesses can be caused by eating or handling contaminated foods, animals, or animal products. Generally speaking, the onset of the symptoms varies from a couple of hours to several days after contact, depending on the nature of the disease.

Specific Diseases

Gastroenteritis Gastroenteritis is caused by drinking contaminated water and/or ingesting food contaminated with staphylococci, *Shigella* bacteria, or other food-borne organisms. Another type of gastroenteritis is giardiasis, one of the most common parasitic diseases among backpackers diagnosed in the United States. This disease can often be transmitted from person to person within a family group or institution. Diarrheal illness, with its potential for significant fluid loss and dehydration, has more serious implications in infants.

Signs The signs vary depending upon the cause and include explosive watery diarrhea at onset, abdominal pains, and vomiting. Periodic bouts of loose stools and a low-grade fever may be present.

Treatment The immediate consideration in the treatment of gastroenteritis is the replacement of water, sodium chloride, potassium, and bicarbonate lost through vomiting and diarrheal stools. For mild cases take broth, carbonated drinks, or Gatorade to replace the fluid loss. Avoid milk or milk products. Diarrheal illnesses cause intolerance for milk sugar (lactose), and ingesting lactose can aggravate or prolong the diarrhea. Fluids taken often and in small amounts are better tolerated than those drunk in large quantity in a short period of time. The Center for Disease Control, Atlanta, Georgia, suggests a home treatment which replaces the lost fluids and electrolytes (see Table 1). The most effective drug to control the symptoms is Pepto-Bismol. The adult dosage is 2 tablespoons every 30 minutes to a maximum of eight doses. More acute cases should be referred to a physician.

Note: When one is traveling in foreign countries where sanitary conditions are suspect, it is safe to drink only hot beverages (coffee or tea) made with boiling water, beer, wine, and canned or bottled carbonated water or beverages. Also, be sure to avoid unpasteurized milk and milk products.

Staphylococcal Food Poisoning (Staph) This is the most common cause of food poisoning. Poisoning may result from eating a variety of foods (meat, poultry, fish, dairy products, custards, and cream-filled pastries) left at room temperature too long. These foods are easily contaminated. They must be properly covered and immediately refrigerated in warm weather.

TABLE 1
Home Treatment for Diarrhea: Prepare One Glass of Each of the Following

Glass No. 1*		Glass No. 2	
8 oz	Orange, apple, or other fruit juice (rich in potassium)	8 oz	Tap water (boiled or carbonated if purity of source unknown)
½ tsp	Honey or corn syrup (rich in glucose necessary for absorption of essential salts)	¼ tsp	Baking soda (sodium bicarbonate)
1 pinch	Table salt (sodium chloride)		

Drink alternately from each glass. Supplement with carbonated beverages, water (boiled if necessary), tea, or coffee if desired.

* Gatorade ingredients are similar to Glass No. 1.

Signs Symptoms occur 2 to 8 hours after ingestion and include nausea, abdominal cramps, diarrhea, headache, and low-grade fever.

Treatment Treatment consists of rapid replacement of fluid, and bed rest. (See "Treatment" under "Gastroenteritis.")

Shigella (Shigellosis or Bacillary Dysentery) Epidemics of shigellosis occur in overcrowded populations with inadequate sanitation. The source of the infection is from the excreta of infected individuals. It is often spread by contaminated food.

Signs The symptoms occur 1 to 4 days after contact. The onset, especially in younger children, is sudden, with fever, irritability or drowsiness, nausea and vomiting, anorexia, diarrhea, and abdominal pain.

Treatment Replacement of fluids and electrolyte loss. (see "Treatment" under "Gastroenteritis.")

Rabies (Hydrophobia) Rabies is an acute infectious disease of animals. Infected wildlife is the major source of human exposure in the United States, as most domesticated animals are vaccinated against rabies. The most commonly infected wild animals include skunks, foxes, raccoons, and bats. If a domesticated animal bites a person, contain the animal for observation. *Do not* kill the animal. Call the Humane Society so the animal can be captured and observed. If it is a wild animal, report the incident to the park ranger or game warden. Small wild animals, except bats, do not normally attack humans unless cornered. All meat-eating animals are susceptible to rabies and are capable of transmitting the infection.

Treatment The wound should be treated as a puncture wound. Wash thoroughly in warm water and soap. Follow with a complete rinse of the wound with water. Apply an antiseptic solution and a dry, sterile dressing. Refer to a physician. Specific follow-up treatment of rabies consists of the administering of a series of vaccine injections. A new vaccine for the treatment of rabies called Wyvac has been developed by the Wyeth Laboratories.[1] It is easier to give, safer to use, and more likely to work (98 percent success rate) than the previous vaccine. It has also reduced the number of doses necessary from 23 to 6. Individuals whose occupation increases their risk of exposure or cave explorers who may be

[1] FDA approval pending.

exposed to bats should probably be vaccinated prophy-lactically.

Tetanus (Lockjaw) Tetanus is an acute infection that may occur in any wound, especially a dirty one. The bacteria are prevalent in the soil and especially in animal feces and excretions. Drug addicts and burn victims are also susceptible to this infection. A tetanus booster shot should be obtained every 10 years. If a serious injury occurs, or if a person is traveling to remote areas, the booster shot should be updated.

Cellulitis Cellulitis is an infection that may result from a wound contaminated with common skin bacteria. It may also occur where there is tissue injury, but no apparent break in the skin. The infection spreads, if unchecked, affecting the skin and underlying tissues. The infection is prone to spread rather easily to other areas if unchecked.

Signs The site of the infection is swollen, red, and warm and tender to touch. Fever, chills, and general body weakness may be present.

Treatment Treatment involves rest and elevation of the involved part. Hot, wet towels should be applied. An antibiotic should be used to control the infection and a physician's services should be obtained.

Allergies People are allergic to many things in the environment. Offending substances include pollen, food, drugs, bacteria, house dust, and pets. Some individuals have an allergic reaction to heat, light, cold, or emotional stress. The most common allergic manifestations are asthma, hay fever, hives, and reactions to certain foods or drugs.

Hay Fever   Hay fever is one of the most common allergic conditions afflicting individuals who are sensitive to ragweed pollen, dust, and other particles in the air. It is most likely to occur in the spring, late summer, and fall months.

Signs   The signs are similar to those for a head cold, including itching and runny nose and sneezing. The eyes are often red, swollen, and watery.

Treatment   Anyone suffering from this condition should probably be under a physician's care. Avoid pollen, dust, and conditions that may aggravate the hay fever. An antihistamine and/or decongestant will offer some relief.

Hives   Hives is an allergic skin reaction caused by the body's sensitivity to various agents. Foods like chocolate, seafood, and fruits such as strawberries and green apples are the worst offenders. Hives may also be caused by the injection of a drug or by emotional stress. Usually this condition is not serious and recovery is complete.

Signs   Large red or white welts resembling insect bites appear. The welts may come and go. Severe itching is usually present.

Treatment   Cornstarch baths or calamine lotion may relieve the itching. Antihistamines will offer some relief. Occasionally, medical assistance and prescription drugs are necessary to treat the more severe cases.

Drug Reactions   Some individuals have mild to severe reactions to certain drugs such as penicillin or aspirin. An overdose of a particular drug or medication that has not been a problem previously may produce a reaction. For most people, medications prescribed by physicians are safe.

Signs   The signs are skin rashes, unexpected fever, shock, and possible altered consciousness.

Treatment   People with drug allergies should consult their physicians to determine the cause of the allergy.

Problems Involving Eyes, Ears, Nose, and Throat

A number of ailments affect the eyes, ears, nose, and throat. As a rule they are seldom disabling. However, some, if untreated, may develop into an upper respiratory problem.

Eye Infections   Two of the most comon eye infections are the sty and pinkeye. A person may also get an infection in the eye as a result of the presence of a foreign object.

Sty (Hordeolum)   A sty is an infection of one of the glands on the edge of the eyelid.
Signs   The eyelid is red, swollen, and inflamed.

Treatment Warm, moist compresses for 20 minutes every 3 hours.

Pinkeye Pinkeye is often transmitted from child to child in school situations and is highly contagious. It is believed to be caused by a virus.

Signs Inflammation and redness of the surface of the eye. A burning and itching sensation in the eye likened to "sand in the eye."

Treatment Apply cold compresses to the eye for relief. Seek medical attention.

Infection from Foreign Object in the Eye Remove the foreign object by rinsing with lukewarm water. Apply warm, moist compresses to the eye. Refer to a physician.

Ear Infections Ear infections often occur with or after a cold or similar type of viral infection. They may also be caused by swimming, a foreign object in the ear, or sometimes, a rapid change in altitude.

Signs Sharp pain in the ear, possible dizziness, fever, and hearing loss. Redness and swelling of the ear canal may be present.

Treatment Apply warm compresses frequently to the ear. Give two aspirin every 4 hours to relieve the pain. Insert a light cotton wad saturated with saline solution into the ear. Seek medical assistance. If an insect is in the ear, use drops of warm mineral or olive oil. This will smother the insect and will give relief from the pain. *Note:* If the ear is draining, it should be kept dry.

Common Cold A large number of viruses cause the common cold and upper respiratory ailments. They are usually spread through person-to-person contact.

Signs Soreness and dryness of the throat, nasal stuffiness, sniffles, and a watery discharge from the nose. A hacking cough may develop. A fever may be present, but the person's temperature is rarely as high as 102°F. It is often stated of the common cold, "As a rule, if the symptoms are treated, it usually will subside in 7 days. If untreated, the symptoms last a week!"

Treatment Treatment consists of rest and drinking lots of fluids, especially citrus juices. Give two aspirin four times daily for fever. Avoid chilling, and decrease activity. Warm saltwater gargles are helpful for the sore throat. A nasal decongestant such as Afrin nasal spray is helpful for a stuffy nose. If cough persists, consult with your physician.

Sore Throat A sore throat is a common symptom. It often accompanies a common cold or the *flu*. A strep throat, laryngitis, pharyngitis, and tonsillitis are more serious infections associated with a sore throat. Continued hoarseness is an important sign of a more serious throat problem.

Signs The throat is red (inflamed) and sore. Fever may be present. Hoarseness, a dry, scratchy feeling in the throat, and perhaps difficulty in talking and swallowing may be present. In some cases, swelling of the lymph nodes of the neck will occur.

Treatment   Use warm saline gargles four times daily (1 teaspoon of salt per glass of water). Drink plenty of fluid, especially citrus juices. Rest and take two aspirin four times daily. Throat lozenges or cough syrup may provide relief. Most sore throats will subside in 3 to 6 days. If symptoms continue or if there is an increase in temperature, consult your physician. A more serious throat infection has probably occurred.

Influenza   Influenza, or the flu, is a viral infection that usually occurs during the winter months. It is spread by person-to-person contact. Vaccinations have been of value in preventing certain types of influenza. In severe cases a more serious illness such as pneumonia may develop.

Signs   These are headache, weakness, muscle aching, loss of appetite, and fatigue. Upper respiratory symptoms including a cough, sore throat, and nasal congestion will be present. The face is warm and flushed. Chilliness and fever up to 102 to 103°F develop. The victim has "aches and pains."

Treatment   Bed rest, warmth, and lack of exertion are recommended. Give lots of fluids, especially citrus juices, and place on a light diet. Give two aspirin every four hours to relieve the pain and fever. Nasal decongestants and warm saltwater gargles are advisable. Seek medical attention if the condition does not respond to treatment.

Sinusitis   Sinusitis is an infection caused by an obstruction of the nasal sinuses. It usually is caused by a cold or an allergy. Mucus collects in the sinus and becomes infected. This infection affects the surrounding tissue, causing swelling and inadequate drainage of the sinus cavity.

Signs The signs are swelling and tenderness around the eyes and nose, and headache and pain, especially behind the eyes. The infection often creates a *post-nasal drip,* which is a drainage of thick, yellow mucus from the nose along the back of the throat. Acute sinusitis, if untreated, can lead to a serious, threatening infection.

Treatment Get plenty of rest and sleep. The use of a decongestant every 4 hours and an antihistamine are of value. Steam inhalations are sometimes effective. If the condition fails to respond to treatment, seek medical advice.

Canker Sores Canker sores are small, painful ulcers that appear inside the mouth or on the lips. The cause is unknown; however, they seem to follow gastric, physical, and emotional stress.

Signs There are small blisters that break, leaving a small white or yellowish sore surrounded by a red halo.

Treatment Increase fluid intake and avoid any acidic food or drinks. Rinse the mouth out four times daily with a solution of baking soda and water or salt and water. Follow with a rinse of 3% hydrogen peroxide solution and water (half and half). An oral suspension of tetracycline may be prescribed. Hold the suspension in the mouth for

2 to 5 minutes and then swallow. It may be given four times daily for 4 days. If sores persist, consult a physician.

Special Medical Problems of Women

Certain medical problems relate only to women, who should be aware of some of the disorders they may encounter. Women should follow the recommended hygienic practices and preventive measures and obtain the necessary medical care. A complete gynecological examination is recommended, including a breast exam and a Pap smear (test for cervical cancer), for all women on a yearly basis, or more frequently if recommended by the physician. Specialists generally suggest that the first examination be done by the age of 17 to 18, at the onset of sexual activity, or earlier if pain or abnormal bleeding develops.

Cystitis Cystitis is an acute urinary tract infection with inflammation of the bladder.

Signs Frequency of urination, urinary urgency, burning on urination or painful urination, possibly with associated low-back pain, and a feeling of inadequate emptying of the bladder are experienced.

Treatment Consult a physician for diagnosis and treatment. A delay in obtaining treatment may result in serious complications.

Preventive Measures Drink lots of fluid; practice good personal hygiene such as washing thoroughly and always wiping from front to back; do not delay going to the bathroom; and always urinate after intercourse.

Vaginitis Vaginitis is an inflammation of the vagina causing a distressing discharge from the genital tract. Some vaginal discharge (whitish, clear to cloudy, and nonbloody) is normal in all women. The amount and consistency differs in individuals at different times during the menstrual cycle.

Signs There is an abnormal white, creamy white, or yellow vaginal discharge characterized by a change in the color, consistency, and odor. The discharge may be accompanied by irritation and/or itching.

Treatment Consult a physician for diagnosis and treatment.

Preventive Measures Practice good personal hygiene and cleanliness and wear cotton underwear, which is more absorbent than synthetic materials. The use of condoms for sexual intercourse helps prevent sexually transmitted disease.

Painful Menstruation and Abnormal Bleeding

Painful Menstruation (Dysmenorrhea) Dysmenorrhea is one of the most common menstrual disorders. It is the greatest single cause of lost working hours and school days among young women. All the causes of dysmenorrhea are not clearly understood, but since it may result from a disease of the pelvis, a physician should be consulted.

Signs Crampy pain over the lower abdomen may radiate to the back and thighs. Some women experience nausea, vomiting, diarrhea, headache, fatigue, nervousness, and dizziness.

Treatment Rest, apply a hot-water bottle to the abdomen, and take aspirin. Consult a physician for evaluation and more extensive care.

Abnormal Bleeding The problem of abnormal or excessive bleeding from the vagina is one of the most common gynecological complaints. The cause may stem from a lesion in the genital area, or it may be a functional disorder of the reproductive organs. Either situation requires investigation by a physician.

Since most women expect a relatively regular menstrual pattern, any deviation from this pattern is often a concern to them. Women should not be hesitant about calling their physician to ask for advice about variations in bleeding patterns.

It should be noted that many women experience changes in their menstrual patterns while they are on wilderness outings because their cycle can be influenced by changes in environment, altitude, climate, and other external factors. Their periods may be late or early, and the quantity of discharge may be different.

The problem that would be of great concern during this time is profuse bleeding. If this occurs and medical assistance is hours away, stop all activity. Lie down with the feet elevated until transportation can be arranged. Do not take aspirin, as it may increase bleeding. Substitute Tylenol or similar medication for relief of pain. Drink ample fluids.

Special Childhood Emergencies

Special understanding is necessary when caring for a child who is ill or has been injured. Your calmness and ability to reassure the child are important in providing the proper care.

Accidents Accidents are the most common cause of injuries and deaths during childhood. They include falls, burns, drownings, suffocation, poisonings, and the swallowing of objects. Most accidents arise from the child's curiosity and are preventable. They occur when the home is the busiest and the child is left unattended. Safety education for the parent is most important in the prevention of the majority of accidents. This information can be obtained from your physician.

Illnesses It is important to understand some of the special illnesses or problems that children encounter. Some of these problems are serious; others are not. If there is any doubt, contact your physician.

- Children are susceptible to many diseases throughout childhood which require immunization during infancy.
- Children are more vulnerable than adults to the stings and bites of poisonous insects, snakes, and marine life.
- Severe vomiting and diarrhea are more dangerous in infants and young children (a higher percentage of their body weight as compared to adults is comprised of fluids).
- Children may vomit without warning, may develop a fever without any obvious reason, or may cry for an indefinite length of time.

Specific Childhood Illnesses

Colic   Colic is characterized by crying and irritability, apparently caused by abdominal pain. Infants may experience this problem shortly after they are brought home from the hospital. It may continue until 3 to 4 months of age. Typically, the colicky infant eats well, gains weight, but has sudden and violent outbursts of crying. Usually colic appears at regular times of the day or night, but in some cases the child cries continuously. Colicky infants are essentially healthy, and this behavior usually ceases in a few weeks. Frequent crying is not necessarily harmful.

Signs   There are sudden and violent outbursts of crying. A strong sucking urge may be present.

Treatment   Infants who cry for short periods of time may respond to holding, rocking, or patting. If a fever or weight loss is present, check with your physician.

Croup   Croup is primarily an infection of the larynx in children between 6 months and 3 years of age, but it may occasionally occur in older children. It is a viral infection that causes severe coughing and noisy breathing and often follows a cold or other infection. The coughing is usually more severe in the evening after the child is in bed. The illness usually lasts 3 to 4 days.

Signs   The signs are a spasmodic or "barking" cough, hoarseness, and swelling of the throat. Attacks may increase the pulse and certainly affect breathing. The child is fatigued.

Treatment Any severe case should be seen by a physician. Rest and warmth for the child is important. The use of a steam vaporizer is valuable. Some relief from symptoms may be gained by holding the child upright over the shoulder for 20 to 30 minutes. Keep the child warm by wrapping him or her in a blanket.

Diarrhea Frequent loose bowel movements occur in all infants. They are not normally considered serious unless associated with vomiting, lack of appetite, weight loss, listlessness, or bloody stools. Breast-fed infants have frequent frothy bowel movements, especially if they are not receiving solid foods. Sudden, or "explosive," diarrhea with the above signs usually indicates an infection is present.

Treatment Refer the child to a physician to determine the cause. A soft, bland diet is advisable.

Acute Infectious Gastroenteritis Infants and children are more likely to have gastroenteritis than older people. In the majority of cases the cause is not determined.

Signs Excessive vomiting, diarrhea, and dehydration (especially in infants under 3 months of age) occur. Diarrhea may be explosive. Other signs include warm, dry skin; fever; weakness; listlessness; and abdominal pain.

Treatment The treatment consists of replacement and maintenance of fluids. The vomiting and diarrhea are usually controlled by treating the infection, if it is identified. Consult your physician. Fluids such as sugar water, apple or grape juice, or soda beverages are helpful. A soft, bland diet and skim milk can be added as symptoms subside. A return to a full diet is often possible in 3 to 4 days.

Chapter 14
Outdoor, Wilderness, and Altitude Problems

In this section a number of medical and altitude problems often encountered in the wilderness will be discussed. Most of the problems result from inadequate preparation, carelessness, or lack of respect for the wilderness. Knowledge concerning the various problems and their proper treatment can prevent most of them from becoming serious.

Sunburn Sunburns are especially likely to occur at altitudes of 3000 feet and above, even if the affected person already has a good tan. Thirty minutes' exposure at this elevation may produce redness of the exposed skin and swelling, especially around the joints. More prolonged exposure on a bright day may cause pain and blistering.

Special preventive steps should be taken when one is climbing at the higher elevations. Reflection of the sun off rocks, light soil, water, or snow can severely burn the eyes and other parts of the body. Important preventive measures include wearing a wide-brim hat, light clothing, a bandana over the neck, and a good pair of sunglasses.

The application of a sunscreen or glacial cream to the ears, under the eyes, nose, etc., will help prevent sunburn.

Treatment Apply a cold, wet dressing soaked in a boric acid solution (1 teaspoon per quart of water), followed by a soothing sunburn cream. Keep out of the sun as much as possible.

Snowblindness Snowblindness or sun blindness is due to excessive exposure of the eyes to the sun. Similar conditions could occur from exposure to an ultraviolet light or electric welding equipment. The symptoms may not occur until several hours after exposure. The best preventive measures are to wear high-quality sunglasses or goggles. The glasses should be worn during bright sunlight and in partly cloudy or overcast conditions. They should be large enough to protect from the sides and below.

Signs The eyes feel dry and irritated, as if they were full of sand (a gritty feeling). Swelling of the eyelids may occur, with burning and redness of the eyes. In severe cases there may be difficulty in seeing. Pain may be severe.

Treatment Apply cold, damp compresses to the eyes and place the person in a dark environment. An hourly application of an ophthalmic ointment will help relieve the pain. The affected person should wear dark glasses and stay out of the sunlight for several days.

Blisters A blister on the foot is one of the most common problems encountered by hikers. Blisters are also caused by burns or by severe pinching (the latter are referred to as *blood blisters*). Most blisters are caused by friction and pinching of the shoe and can be avoided. Important preventive measures include getting your feet in good condition prior to long hiking trips; wearing properly fitted and *well-broken-in* boots; and wearing light cotton socks under heavy wool socks. Usually the affected area on the foot becomes warm and develops what is known as a *hot spot* from the friction created inside the boot. If this occurs, the person should stop and place a piece of adhesive tape over the area as a buffer. This padding will assist in preventing a blister. If a blister appears, make a doughnut out of moleskin (see Figure 1). Place the moleskin around the blister and secure it with adhesive tape.

Signs The area becomes warm and a hot spot develops; some redness and tenderness will be present. Swelling occurs, with either white fluid or blood under the skin.

Treatment Ordinarily a blister should not be opened because of the risk of infection. If it is necessary, because of certain activities (walking, using the hand), to open the blister:

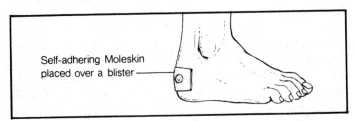

Self-adhering Moleskin
placed over a blister —

Figure 1 Applying moleskin over a hot spot or a blister.

- Wash the area thoroughly with soap and water.
- Insert a sterilized needle under the edge of the blister on each side.
- Press down on the fluid or blood, forcing it out through the tiny openings.
- Apply a mild antiseptic to the area.
- Apply a Telfa sterile pad and a DSD.

If the blister has ruptured, treat as an abrasion. Keep it clean to prevent infection. If the skin flap causes irritation, it should be cut off and a DSD and a moleskin doughnut applied (see Figure 1).

Chafing (Intertrigo) Chafing is a condition usually associated with hot weather, perspiration, and hiking, especially with heavier people. It occurs where the moist skin rubs together, e.g., between the thighs, between the cheeks of the buttocks, or under the breasts. *Diaper rash* is also a form of intertrigo.

Treatment Wash the area thoroughly with warm water and soap, and dry thoroughly. Apply a talc powder liberally three to four times daily to the area. Wear clean cotton undergarments and limit physical activity during hot weather.

Cold Sores (Herpes Simplex) Cold sores or *fever blisters* are caused by a virus and can be triggered by the unfiltered ultraviolet light of the sun. They usually occur around the mouth and lips. Gradual exposure to the sun and the liberal use of a sunscreen or glacial cream on the face and lips are good preventive measures. A medicated lip balm or Labiosan topical protectant is helpful in prevention.

Signs   Small blisters or sores appear around the mouth and lips.

Treatment   Keep the area clean. Apply tincture of benzoin, or use a soothing topical protectant anesthetic ointment such as Labiosan.

Constipation   Constipation is the presence of hard stools, often associated with difficulty in passage and/or infrequency of bowel movement. It may result from a disruption of the normal daily routine, a change in the diet, and a reduced fluid intake. It is not uncommon to have a bowel movement only every 2 to 3 days in the wilderness. The most important preventive measures include drinking lots of fluids (at least 2 quarts a day) and eating plenty of roughage, fruits, and vegetables.

Treatment   If condition persists, a dose of mineral oil or a mild laxative will normally relieve the problem.

Dehydration   Dehydration is a condition that results when an excessive amount of water or fluid is lost from the body. It may be caused by sweating, excessive vomiting, diarrhea, or evaporation of fluids from the lungs. It can be caused by insufficient intake of water and salt, illness, fever, hot weather, high altitudes, and/or vigorous activities. The average amount of fluids a person needs daily is 2 to 3 quarts. This amount should be increased to 6 to 8 quarts under certain conditions. The body also needs 3 to 5 grams of salt daily. (Salt aids in the body's retention of fluids.) If excessive perspiration or fluid loss occurs, this amount may be increased to 15 grams a day. This water and salt balance is a *must* in the prevention of dehydration.

Perhaps the best signal of fluid imbalance within the body is the *urine spot test*. This is referred to as the *snow flowers*. If someone urinates in the snow, the color will usually be light yellow. If the person becomes dehydrated, it will turn to a dark brownish orange color.

Signs The signs are extreme thirst, dark yellow to brownish orange urine, and gradual or sudden cessation of urination. Other symptoms may include headache, dizziness, a very dry cotton-mouth sensation, difficulty in speaking coherently, a tired or lazy feeling, loss of appetite, nausea, drowsiness, and fever.

Treatment Treatment for dehydration includes avoidance of energy loss and replacement of fluids and salt. Get the victim out of the hot environment and into the shade. A seriously dehydrated person will have little appetite and must be urged to drink small quantities of fluids (with salt and sugar) at frequent intervals. As a rule, double the normal fluid intake for the particular environment you are in. Individuals who are seriously dehydrated are in need of medical assistance.

Methods of Conserving Energy and Preventing Dehydration

- Drink all the water you need, especially when thirsty.
- Drink water at regular intervals.
- Drink water while eating; eat regular, lighter meals even if not hungry.

- Nibble food continuously, especially food with a high salt and sugar content.
- Drink warm liquids and supplement the diet, especially in cold climate.
- Be in good physical condition prior to starting a trip.
- Slow down the activity in hot weather; get plenty of rest (5 to 10 minutes' rest each hour).
- Wear proper clothing in both hot and cold environments.
- Keep dry, carry lighter loads, and avoid excessive perspiration.
- Stay comfortable in both warm and cold weather.
- Travel at times when it is not as hot; seek the shade.
- Do not smoke, do not drink alcoholic beverages, cut down on conversation.
- Most important, carefully ration your water.

Diarrhea (Trots)   Diarrhea is a problem frequently encountered in the wilderness or in foreign travel. The change in surroundings, eating contaminated food, drinking contaminated water, the *stomach flu,* and psychological stress are the most common causes. Traveler's diarrhea is referred to as *Montezuma's revenge, turista, the Aztec two-step,* and *backpacker's diarrhea.* Under normal conditions and with proper treatment, diarrhea can be easily controlled. Severe diarrhea, the cause of which is most frequently transmitted by contaminated drinking water, may lead to dehydration and shock. This is a severe medical emergency. To prevent diarrhea:

- Purify the water by boiling, using iodine crystals or purification tablets (see "Nutrition: Foraging for Food and Water" in Chapter 19).

- Do not eat food that you are not sure about (the water in certain foods may be contaminated).

- Use your own dishes (we can tolerate our own "bugs" or bacteria but not others').

- Thoroughly cleanse your dishes after use. Use the three-bucket technique of (1) washing in hot water and soap, (2) use of a disinfectant rinse, and (3) end with a cold-water rinse.

Signs The signs are frequent, loose, and watery stools, often accompanied by nausea, vomiting, and abdominal cramps.

Treatment Stop activity and obtain rest. Fluids that contain salt and sugar, e.g., Gatorade thirst quencher, weak tea, broth, and soups are recommended. Medications such as Pepto-Bismol upset stomach remedy or Lomotil every 4 hours may help relieve the diarrhea (see "Treatment" under "Gastroenteritis" in Chapter 13).

Carbon Monoxide Poisoning The traveler should take special precautionary steps to prevent carbon monoxide poisoning by:

- Never burning an open-flame heater or lantern in an enclosed space without proper ventilation.

- Never using catalytic heaters which can be dangerous in campers and trailers.

- Keeping the windows partly open for cross ventilation in automobiles.

- Keeping the exhaust free from any snow.

Signs The signs are headache, dizziness, difficulty in breathing, drowsiness, and later unconsciousness.

Treatment Get the victim into fresh air. Provide BCLS if necessary.

Wounds and Injuries in the Wilderness

The most common serious injury occurring in the wilderness is a cut. Cuts are usually caused by hand tools such as knives and axes. Other frequent injuries include sprains, strain, bruises, and fractures.

There is no special care necessary in the treatment of most injuries in the wilderness. Use the same basic wound-management techniques described in Chapter 5, "Wounds and Related Injuries." Good judgment must be exercised in determining whether an injured person should continue the trip and what means of transportation should be provided a seriously injured person.

With respect to open wounds, there is an increased danger of infection if proper treatment and cleanliness are not provided. Initially, the bleeding should be controlled by a direct-pressure bandage, using the cleanest available material. Generally speaking, after the bleeding has been controlled, the wound should be cleansed thoroughly. Most wounds will stop bleeding in 6 to 10 minutes under normal conditions. To treat wounds in the wilderness:

- Cleanse the wound with warm water and a mild soap (boil the water and allow it to cool before cleansing the wound, to prevent contamination). Cleanse daily to help prevent infection.

- Always wash away from the wound while cleansing.
- Remove any small objects in the wound with tweezers (deeply embedded objects should not be removed).
- Do not apply creams or salves, as they will keep the wound moist and promote infection.
- Use butterfly bandages to close the wound if necessary.
- Place a Telfa sterile pad over the wound to keep the bandage from sticking, or secure with a dry, sterile dressing. Keep the bandage open at the sides to allow the wound to scab over.
- If there is danger of the wound becoming soiled or wet, completely cover the wound with DSD and cover with a light plastic.

All large or serious wounds should be referred to a medical facility after the bleeding has been controlled. Normally, do not rebandage the wound unless medical help will be unavailable for several days. If help is unavailable, the wound should be cleansed at a time when there is no danger of further bleeding. This time span may range from 30 minutes to several hours. Provide basic wound management (see Chapter 5) and refer to a medical facility as soon as possible. Cleanliness is of primary importance for the prevention of infection. Treat any individual with a serious wound for shock.

If a wound becomes infected, soak it in warm water (after boiling the water) for 15 to 20 minutes three to four times daily. The water should be as warm as the person can tolerate. After soaking the infected part, place it in a position of complete rest. The person should remain quiet and plans should be made to evacuate. An antibiotic such as penicillin is usually necessary to control infection. For other medically related problems occurring in the wilderness, use the standard treatment indicated in other sections of the guide. Your greatest responsibility after treating the injury or ailment is to determine whether the person should be referred to a medical facility and which method of evacuation should be used. *Take your time. Make a sound and logical decision.*

Altitude Problems

The major problems at high altitudes are *acute mountain sickness* (AMS), *high-altitude pulmonary edema* (HAPE), and *cerebral edema* (CE). In climbing to elevations of 3000 feet and above, the body needs to make certain physiological adaptations, and this takes time. This adaptation is referred to as *acclimatization*. Achieving acclimatization requires continuous exposure at the increased elevation. The most noticeable changes taking place within the body during acclimatization are:

- An increase in the respiratory rate (ventilation), causing an undue shortness of breath.

- An elevation of pressure in the pulmonary arteries which increases the capacity of the lung to absorb oxygen (O_2).

- An increase in the number of red blood cells (RBCs). This increase permits the blood to carry more O_2 at higher elevations (RBCs carry O_2). An increase in the RBCs also allows an easier release of O_2 to the tissues.

- An increased cardiac output during the first few days at higher elevations.

Generally it takes approximately 10 days for the circulatory and respiratory adaptations to take place. The increase in RBCs reaches approximately 80 percent in 10 days and acclimatization is nearly complete in 6 weeks.

The best way to achieve proper acclimatization to higher altitudes is to have minimal activity during the first 4 days. As you are climbing, ascend 500 to 1000 feet daily, depending upon the amount of physical exertion expended, with frequent rest stops. The best way to prevent altitude sickness is to take time for the climb. Here are some general principles regarding altitude sickness:

- Strenuous exertion increases the risk of altitude problems.
- Frequent rests are necessary to allow the body to gradually adjust to the higher altitudes.
- Good physical condition appears to offer little protection.
- Children appear to be more vulnerable than adults (normally they are more active).
- Men and women appear equally susceptible (it is possible that women may have a greater risk during the week prior to menstruation).
- A person who has had one attack of altitude sickness may be more likely to have another.
- A person is more likely to develop HAPE if he or she descends after adapting to an altitude and then returns within a few days or weeks (acclimatization is lost in about a week after returning to sea level).
- The use or increase of special vitamins does not appear to be of any value.
- If any warning signs of altitude sickness appear, *descend.*

For altitude sickness, medication, treatment, and oxygen are *not* substitutes for descending to richer oxygen supplies found at the lower altitudes.

Acute Mountain Sickness (AMS) Acute mountain sickness is a condition that occurs at higher elevations, commonly above the 7000- to 8000-foot level. It is primarily due to the lack of O_2 in the system (blood and brain). An individual who climbs too quickly to a higher elevation may experience difficulty in breathing and an increase in pulse rate. There may be a decrease in appetite and difficulty in sleeping. The climber should avoid heavy foods and favor a liquid diet. Usually in a few days the appetite returns. Climbers should not overexert themselves during the first 4 days of the climb. Avoid smoking and drinking strong coffee or alcoholic beverages.

Signs Headaches, dizziness, nausea, vomiting, loss of appetite, increase in pulse rate, shortness of breath, and sleeping problems are experienced.

Treatment Rest and only light activity are recommended. Give fluids (water, tea, soups, etc.) and a light diet. Aspirin for the headache and a mild sedative (phenobarbital) may be prescribed to promote sleep. Sleeping at lower altitude often helps, but descent is usually unnecessary. A mild diuretic, such as Diamox, may have some value in minimizing AMS; however, it must be taken several days before and during the ascent. It is not a substitute for time. AMS usually improves in 1 to 2 days if the person drinks plenty of liquids, takes aspirin, and remains mildly active. Encourage deep breathing and give oxygen if available. Individuals who continue vomiting must descend.

High-Altitude Pulmonary Edema (HAPE) High-altitude pulmonary edema is a condition that usually occurs above the 10,000-foot level. It may develop below this level if the person is overly active upon arrival. It results from ascending too rapidly and is a serious medical emergency. The causes of HAPE are not clearly understood. There appears to be a leakage of fluid from the small blood vessels in the lungs, allowing this fluid to seep into the air sacs (alveoli). As the fluids accumulate in the air sacs, the transfer of oxygen and carbon dioxide between the blood and lungs is seriously impaired. HAPE may cause death by drowning from excess water in the lungs.

Signs The symptoms of AMS are present, along with a dry, hacking cough. Undue shortness of breath develops with a tightness in the chest. Weakness, extreme fatigue, and a feeling of suffocation during sleep will be experienced. Later the cough will bring up a watery and frothy liquid which may be pink with blood. Abnormal sounds can be heard in the chest. As the condition worsens, the lips and nail beds may turn blue with the victim becoming pale and cold. Loss of mental acuity (sharpness) and unconsciousness may develop.

Treatment Upon development of any signs of HAPE, the golden rule is to descend. A descent of 2000 to 3000 feet may improve the person's condition. Do not allow the person to continue climbing, even if all the signs disappear. All serious cases should be evacuated by stretcher to a hospital. Administer O_2, if available, for 6 to 12 hours. A diuretic, such as Diamox[1] or Lasix, may be of value; however, a diuretic is to be administered only by a physician. HAPE is a serious medical emergency and descent is always the best treatment. Provide BCLS if necessary.

Cerebral Edema (CE) Cerebral edema is a rare condition which normally does not occur below 12,000 feet. An accumulation of excessive water in the brain causes cerebral edema. This may result in permanent brain damage.

Signs The signs are intense, throbbing headache; weakness; double vision; difficulty in walking and using the hands; loss of mental acuity; confusion, memory loss, hallucinations, and psychotic behavior; and sleepiness, possible unconsciousness, and coma.

Treatment Descent is imperative. Evacuate by litter and helicopter. The victim needs immediate hospitalization. Provide BCLS if necessary.

Hyperventilation Hyperventilation is an abnormal breathing pattern. It is often brought on by extreme anxieties, fear, or exposure. Deep respiration at an increased rate causes a depletion of the carbon dioxide in the blood. Individuals who are nervous, tense, or apprehensive are most likely to develop this condition.

Signs A feeling of shortness of breath, rapid pulse, and dizziness is experienced, along with a numbness and

[1] FDA approval pending.

tingling sensation around the mouth, fingers, and toes. Trembling, lightheadedness, and fainting may occur. Muscle spasms may frighten the person even more, compounding the anxiety and causing the victim to breathe even more rapidly.

Treatment Help the person slow down the rapid breathing by offering reassurance and explaining the problem. Have the victim breathe gently into a large paper bag. This allows the person to rebreathe carbon dioxide and reestablish proper oxygen–carbon dioxide balance.

Cheyne-Stokes Respiration Cheyne-Stokes respiration is probably caused by poor cerebral circulation and therefore a deficiency of oxygen to the brain. It refers to a pattern of respiration where the person begins with shallow breathing, increasing in crescendo fashion to deep respirations. Then respiration may even stop for a few seconds. The shallow breaths will resume and the sequence will be continued. This type of breathing may occur at the higher elevations (above 13,000 feet).

Signs The signs are irregular breathing, restlessness, and a feeling of suffocation, especially when awakening from sleep.

Treatment If this type of breathing follows a serious injury, particularly a head injury, it indicates a serious medical emergency and evacuation is imperative.

Chapter 15
Carries and Short-Distance Transfers

After most accidents there are few reasons to move a seriously injured person from his or her present location. Generally speaking, more harm is done through improper movement and transportation than by any other means. In most instances, the seriously injured person should not be moved if professional rescue personnel are available. These highly trained crews have the know-how and the equipment best suited to handle most emergencies. There are times, however, when it is necessary to move a seriously injured person from a life-threatening situation or dangerous location to a place of safety. Examples include the danger of an explosion or fire in the home or in an automobile; the risk of drowning or suffocation; or a serious traffic hazard which may jeopardize the lives of victim and rescuer.

There will be other occasions when you can assist a less seriously injured person to safety or to a medical facility. Knowledge of a few simple carries and short-distance transfers will enable you to provide this person with the needed care.

If you have to make the decision to transport a

seriously injured person, you will need to prepare your equipment and assistants for the task. Initially, however, you should make a complete assessment of the victim's condition and then decide on the method of transfer. In many instances it is necessary to transport the victim in the position he or she is found in, whether on the face, on the back, or on the side. Follow these additional steps and reminders prior to any movement of the victim:

- Anyone with altered consciousness and multiple injuries must be assumed to have spinal injuries.
- Treat all injuries prior to attempting any lift or movement of the injured person.
- Protect the injuries by immobilizing the injured parts.
- Treat the person for shock.
- Make the victim as comfortable as possible. Be reassuring and explain how you will make the move.
- Prepare your equipment (litter, stretcher, backboard) for the carry. Remember, all suspected spine injuries should be transported on a backboard or spinal board.
- Usually transport the seriously injured person in a supine position.
- Practice the lift (on another person) prior to the move. Assistants must be instructed in every detail concerning their role during the lift.
- Carry out the lift in a very slow and methodical manner.

The technique used to transfer the injured person depends upon the nature of the accident, the strength of the rescuer, the number of assistants, and the equipment available. Most carries and transfers require practice, time, and planning to be carried out successfully. Other rescues may necessitate a quick response, such as pulling a person from a burning automobile or carrying a child from a smoke-filled room.

Carries and Transfers

Shoulder Carry The shoulder carry may be used in removing an unconscious person from the water or from a burning building (when neck or spinal injuries are not suspected). Insert your arm in the person's crotch, bringing the chest across your shoulder. Grasp the victim's arm over your opposite shoulder. One hand can easily hold the person's legs securely by grasping the wrist. This will free the opposite hand during the rescue. Care must be exercised during the lift. Squat to one knee, pull the victim onto your back, and lift with the strong muscles of the legs (see Figure 1).

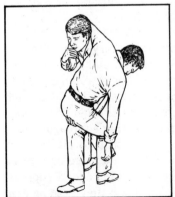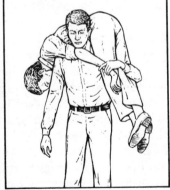

Figure 1 The shoulder or fireman's carry.

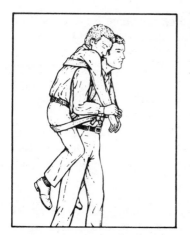

Figure 2 The back carry, or modified pack-strap carry.

Back Carry The single-person back carry or *piggyback carry* is an especially good method for transporting a smaller person with minor injuries for a short distance. There are several variations: with the rescuer holding onto the victim's knees or with the injured person seated in a strap or a rope (see Figure 2).

Two-Person Carry The two-person carry is an excellent technique for carrying a person with minor injuries. The rescuers should be of approximately the same size to provide a smooth carry. Standing side by side, each should place the adjacent arm over the other's shoulder. With the opposite arm, grasp each other's forearm below the elbow. Kneel and allow the victim to sit on your forearms (see Figure 3). The victim can place both arms around the shoulders of the rescuers for added support. *Note:* Rescuers may reverse positions if they become arm weary.

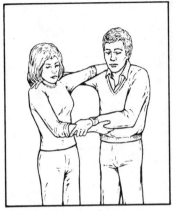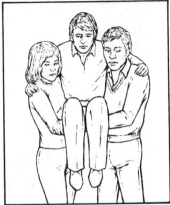

Figure 3 The two-person carry.

Placing a Blanket under the Victim The placement of a blanket under a victim from the side for treatment against shock and minor injuries (assuming no neck or spinal injuries exist) is a relatively easy procedure (see Figure 4). Fold approximately one-half of the blanket lengthwise, placing the pleats along the side of the victim away from you. Elevate the victim's near arm to a bent position. Roll the person toward your lap on the bent-arm side; supporting the body, move the folds or pleats of the blanket in close to the victim's body. In the same manner, reverse this position by rolling the victim to the opposite side onto the blanket. Smooth out the folds and wrap the person in the blanket.

Blanket Drag The blanket drag can be used to remove a heavy person from an area such as a smoke-filled room. You may not have the time to place the blanket

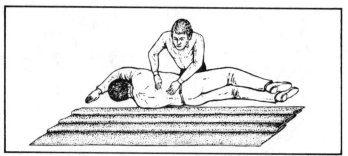

Figure 4 Placing a blanket under a victim from the side position.

under the victim. If this is the case, and assuming no major injuries are present, roll the person quickly onto an open blanket. Wrap the blanket around the victim. Next, lift the head and back off the ground to reduce the friction of the body during the drag. Provide as much protection to the head and neck as possible. Pull with the strong muscles of your legs (see Figure 5). With a heavier victim, two people may be needed to execute the drag. *Note:* Always pull the victim with his or her head and shoulders in the forward position. Do not twist or bend the victim's head, neck, or body during the move.

Litter Transfers In transferring the more seriously injured, there should not be any unnecessary movement of the victim. These techniques should be rehearsed several times prior to the transfer so that all assistants are fully aware of their assignments. Techniques include the traction-blanket insert with lift, the lateral slide onto a litter, and a variation of these transfers.

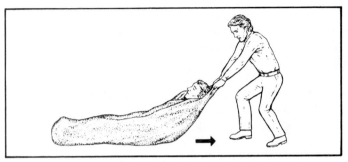

Figure 5 The blanket drag.

Traction-Blanket Insert and Lift   This transfer is made in two separate stages, first the blanket insert and second the lift onto a litter, stretcher, or backboard. Fold a blanket with six folds and place it near the head of the victim. Center the blanket and position it so that it will unfold to its maximum length. The person in charge of the rescue (rescuer 1) should place his or her knee on the end fold of the blanket. The blanket will be pulled under the victim's body in three separate stages. In the first maneuver the blanket will be pulled to the small of the back, then to the knees, and finally past the foot. The person in charge of the rescue will give all instructions and commands during the transfer.

Follow these instructions:

Step One (Blanket Insert)

- First, fold the victim's arms over the chest and bring the feet together.
- The rescuer in charge (rescuer 1) should cradle the victim's

skull with both hands. The rescuer must apply a firm, gentle pressure called *traction* to the head, and maintain this traction during the entire maneuver.

- On command, assistants 2 and 3 insert their hands under, and lift, the victim's shoulders approximately 1 inch off of the ground. Rescuer 1, cradling the head, should elevate the head the same height.

- Assistants 4 and 5 will pull the blanket under the hands of assistants 2 and 3 to the lower part of the victim's back. The blanket slides under the victim's head during this maneuver.

- The assistants repeat this procedure at the hips and at the ankles until the entire blanket has been unfolded under the victim (see Figure 6).

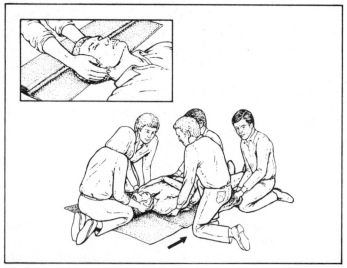

Figure 6   Accordion blanket insertion with traction applied to head.

- *Remember,* maintain traction to the head during the entire maneuver.

Step Two (*Blanket Lift*)

- The assistants roll the blanket up tightly at the sides of the victim.
- The blanket is held with a forward grasp by the assistants.
- Assistants 2 and 4 position their hands at the shoulders and hips, and hips and ankles, respectively. Assistants 3 and 5 align to the opposite side of the victim, placing the hands in the same position.
- On command, the assistants should rock their bodies back to the perpendicular position, keeping their arms straight. *Do not lift.* This will elevate the victim high enough for assistant 6 to slide a litter under the victim from the foot position (see Figure 7). (It is only necessary to elevate the victim to a height sufficient to clear the litter.)

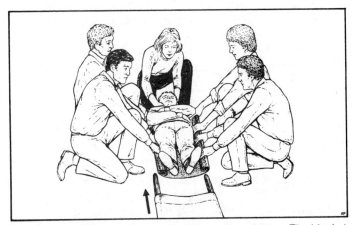

Figure 7 The traction-blanket lift and insertion of litter. The blanket lift can also be used to move the victim found lying in a prone position.

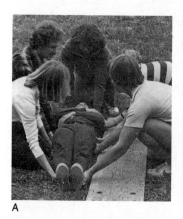 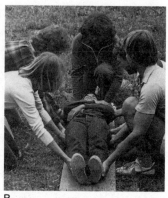

A   B

Figure 8 (a) The lateral-slide technique to move a victim onto a stretcher. (b) Maintain continuous traction to head during move. (*Photo courtesy of Steve Mitgang.*)

- Rescuer 1 maintains traction and support of the head, elevating the victim's head to the same height as the rest of the body during the move. It is important to support the victim's head and neck at all times during the maneuver.
- Lower the victim gently onto the litter and wrap securely in the blanket.
- Immobilize the victim to the litter prior to transportation (see "Fracture of the Neck or Back" in Chapter 7).

The Lateral-Slide Transfer The slide transfer is an alternative method of transferring a seriously injured person onto a litter (see Figure 8). This technique was commonly used by medics before the introduction of the scoop stretcher. The slide transfer requires a minimum of five people. Additional assistants must be employed with heavier victims. The rescuer in charge always maintains the victim's head position and gives the instructions. Place the litter, covered with a blanket, along the side of the victim. Fold the victim's arms over the chest and bring the feet together prior to the transfer. Follow these instructions:

- The strongest assistants, 3 and 5, are on the side reaching across the litter. *Do not kneel on the litter*.

- Assistants 2 and 4 take a similar position on the opposite side of the victim.

- The victim needs to be lifted only as high as the litter (1 to 2 inches).

- Assistants 3 and 5 insert their hands under the edge of the victim's shoulders and hips, and the victim's hips and ankles, respectively. They will lift on command only to a height that clears the edge of the litter.

- Assistants 2 and 4 will place their hands at the same position on the opposite side of the victim. They gently lift and push the victim on command.

- Rescuer 1 gives the command, and *in slow motion* the assistants move the victim very gently. Rescuer 1, maintaining traction to the victim's head, slides laterally, keeping the victim's head and neck in a straight alignment with the victim's body.

- *Note:* If additional assistants are available, position them at the shoulders, hips, and lower legs (three to a side). With an extremely heavy person, it may be necessary to assist by lifting on the belt and the shirt during the maneuver.

Caution: Instruct the assistants never to step over the victim. Always move around the person during the transfer.

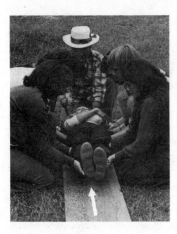

Figure 9 The straight-lift transfer requires at least seven rescuers plus one person to slide the litter under the victim. (*Photo courtesy of Steven Mitgang.*)

Straight-Lift Transfer The straight-lift technique is a variation of the slide transfer and usually calls for seven to nine assistants (depending upon the size of the victim). The person in charge maintains the head position. The assistants kneel along the side of the victim (three or four on each side). They insert their hands under the victim's shoulders, chest, hips, and lower legs. The lift is made upon command, to a height necessary to insert the litter from the foot position (see Figure 9). Gently lower the victim onto the litter and immobilize. If the victim is lying in a prone position, the arms are placed to the side during the lift. The person in charge maintains head traction by supporting the jaw and the side of the head during the lift. *Bear in mind that the heaviest parts of the body are the chest and the hips, so they demand the greatest support.*

Stretchers and Litters

The ideal litter or stretcher for moving a seriously injured person is called the *scoop stretcher*. The scoop is divided into halves. It can be opened, slid under the victim from each side, and locked securely in place (see Figure 10*a*). This maneuver requires very little movement of the injured person during its placement. The Stokes basket stretcher has been used extensively for air-sea rescues in evacuating the seriously injured (see Figure 10*b*). The basket should be lined with a blanket to provide easy

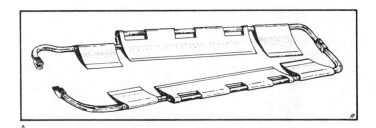

A

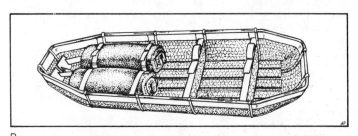

B

Figure 10 (*a*) The split-frame scoop stretcher used by most rescue teams. (*b*) The Stokes basket stretcher. Extremely useful in removing victims from rough terrain.

removal of the victim. The injured person is removed at the emergency room by grasping and lifting the rolled-up blanket at the sides. A new model of the basket stretcher is especially effective for rescue operations as it can accommodate the scoop stretcher and has molded-in runners facilitating removal of the victim over rough terrain. The use of these stretchers permits a safer transfer of the seriously injured.

Improvised Litter If you make the decision to evacuate a seriously injured person, it is usually necessary to improvise the litter. Litters can be made from surfboards, backpack frames, blankets, water skis, or lightweight boards lashed together. A simple blanket-and-pole litter can be improvised by folding a blanket over two 6- to 7-foot poles or green saplings (see Figure 11). The blanket is doubled over with one pole in the folded edge. Next, fold both the edges over the second pole and back over the first. Once this makeshift litter is completed, test it to be sure it is sturdy enough to support the victim. The victim is then placed on the litter so the body lies on the free edge of the blanket, holding it securely in place.

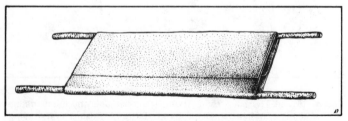

Figure 11 An improvised litter from two green sticks and a blanket.

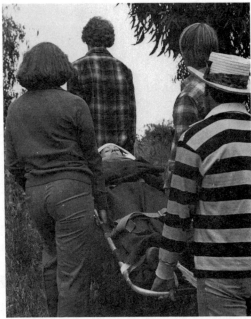

Figure 12 Transporting the litter. Make sure the victim is securely tied to the stretcher. (*Photo courtesy of Steve Mitgang.*)

Completely immobilize the victim. It is especially important to pad the neck and the head during the transfer.

Transporting the Litter During the carry it is recommended that the litter bearers be of approximately the same size, especially in terms of the distance of hands from the ground. This will allow for a smooth and even carry. A minimum of four bearers is usually necessary, two at each end or one at each end and one each on the sides (see Figure 12).

Note: To carry a heavier person and to support an improvised litter you will need six bearers, two at each end and one each at the sides. There is no set rule concerning the position of the victim, other than that the person be carried faceup, unless physical conditions preclude this position. Whether the victim lies in a headfirst or feetfirst position depends upon the nature of the accident and the slant of the terrain. For example, keep the head slightly elevated if head and/or chest injuries are present. If there are injuries to the lower extremities, then the legs should be slightly elevated. The victim's position is often determined by whether you are carrying the person uphill or downhill. Generally speaking, the carry with the head forward on the litter is less frightening to the victim. The exception, however, is in traveling up or down a steep incline, in which case the head should remain elevated.

In summary, it is recommended that the seriously injured be moved by qualified rescue personnel who have both the expertise and equipment to make a safe transfer. However, if it is absolutely necessary to move a person because his or her present position poses a threat to safety, then thoroughly prepare your equipment and assistants for the task. *Remember, the safety and possibly the life of the victim is in your hands.*

Part 2
Outdoor Reference

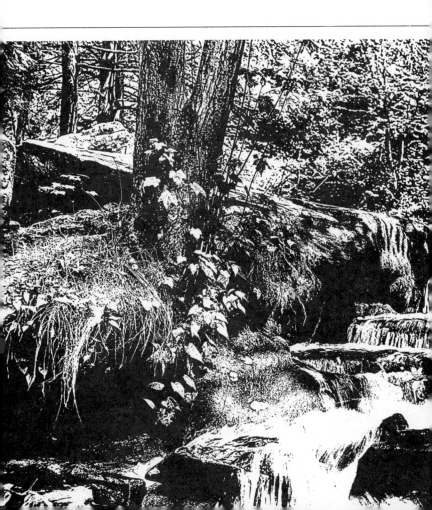

The Wilderness

No one in history has extolled the wilderness more than John Muir. He valued the wilderness as an environment of undisturbed harmony. He said, "No one can be lonesome when everything is wild and beautiful . . . However some have strange morbid fears as soon as they find themselves with Nature, even in the kindest and wildest of her solitudes."

The wilderness is often defined as a forest, a mountainous area, or a desert. It may also designate the sea, a tract of land, or other nonhuman environment where animals are assumed to be present and man is absent.

What the wilderness is to one person may be something entirely different to another. For example, the Hudson Bay trapper would consider a trip to Michigan's Upper Peninsula a return to civilization, while for the vacationer from Los Angeles it indeed may be a wilderness experience. Being caught in a blizzard in Wyoming, capsizing your boat on Lake Michigan, or being forced to land your plane in a nonaccessible place all have wilderness overtones. In essence, the wilderness may be anyplace outdoors in which a person is bewildered, lost, and stripped of his or her guidance.[1]

This section of the guide will help you deal with problems encountered while in the outdoors or what many may call the wilderness. I would like to thank Orrin and Cindy Sage, who acted as advisors in the writing of this section of the guide.

[1] These introductory paragraphs adapted from Roderick Nash, *Wilderness and the American Mind,* rev. ed., Yale University Press, New Haven, Conn., 1973.

Chapter 16

Introduction to the Outdoors

People who travel into the outdoors on an afternoon hike, fly an airplane, go camping, or undertake an extended wilderness outing should expect to find themselves at some time in an emergency situation. Emergencies vary from serious injury to being caught in a sudden storm or becoming lost. To develop rational solutions to various predicaments, you must remain calm and exercise good judgment and common sense. To deal with the unexpected emergency, you must be prepared, patient, and cautious. Your successful handling of any emergency will require both physical and mental preparedness. Well-trained individuals fare much better under adverse conditions and in unexpected situations than those who are unprepared.

Physical Preparedness

Naturally, survival problems are not planned, but you can prepare yourself in advance by being in good physical condition and having the essential equipment, supplies, and skills to deal with emergencies when they happen. Reading books, completing training programs, and combining this knowledge with your own experience prove invaluable when dealing with the unforeseen. Developing specific wilderness skills such as how to use a compass, how to read a topographical map, and how to make a temporary shelter is a necessity. As you enter an unfamiliar area, you should be alert to the surroundings. You should frequently check your location on the map, observe weather conditions, and identify the natural shelters. Alertness will increase your safety by giving you alternative choices for making emergency decisions and will add to your enjoyment of the outdoors.

To be safe, a minimum of four persons should travel together into remote areas. If a serious emergency occurs, this permits one to stay with the victim and two to go for help. The more you decrease the size of your party, the greater the odds are against a safe return. The risks are compounded by the remoteness of the area, inclement weather conditions, and the lack of knowledge and experience. Other considerations upon entering the outdoors and wilderness are:

- Choose your traveling companions carefully. Have knowledge of their capabilities, limitations, and mental attitudes.

- Be sure that all travelers have proper clothing, equipment, and supplies.

- Develop a trip plan—destination, travel routes, time schedule (departure and return); leave this information (with names, addresses, and phone numbers of all members in the party, and automobile color, brand and model, license number, and location) with responsible individuals.

- Consider weather conditions past, present, and future; watch for signals of change.
- Study recent topographical maps, have knowledge of the trails and campsites, and check with authorities for any possible trail changes.
- Know how to use a compass.
- Sign out with proper authorities, forest service, or ranger, and keep them advised if any changes in plans are made; in unscheduled areas, leave a trip plan visible in the window of your automobile.
- Acquire a fire and/or camping permit, and any other permit necessary for the area.
- Plan for delays, advise responsible people of this possibility, and in the event it happens, instruct them in the proper course of action.
- Know the proper emergency signals and how to use them (three of anything: whistle blasts, flares, fires, mirror flashes, etc.).
- Have knowledge of communication and emergency-rescue resources, transportation, and facilities for evacuation and assistance, e.g., sheriff's office, forest service, search and rescue, and the helicopter of the U.S. Coast Guard.
- Put all reports in writing when going for help: include the exact location and nature of the accident, a map, and a possible landing site for a helicopter.

Before venturing into the outdoors or wilderness area, you should plan your program carefully and review the plans for your trip. It is important to select a group leader to coordinate the trip and to see that all in the group are properly prepared. Experience and knowledge are obvious prerequisites for the person who assumes leadership responsibilities. The leader should be able to delegate tasks, utilizing the skills and talents of other members of the group. The group leader must be a strong decision maker but still show sensitivity to the needs of each person in the group, and should have knowledge and understanding of each person's abilities, limitations, and experience. One of the most important attributes of a group leader should be the ability to make logical decisions and resolve problems before they get out of hand. The group leader should be able to anticipate these problems and develop the necessary solutions. In essence, the leader is the one who promotes and provides an enjoyable outing by developing good camping and hiking guidelines for the group. These guidelines should include the following:

- Campers should be able to select their own tentmates, subject to change if conflicts arise. To avoid conflicts, individuals near the same age, mental maturity, and interests are best suited as companions.

- All campers, including the leader, must respect the individual rights and property of others.

- For health purposes, personal cleanliness and good personal hygiene must be practiced at all times.

- It is the responsibility of all members to share in the various duties and chores about the camp. These duties should be rotated as much as possible.

- Be tolerant and considerate of others. For example, proceed only as fast as the slowest member of the party is able to hike.

- Avoid fatigue by moving at a leisurely pace and making frequent rest stops; carefully observe children and inexperienced hikers, as they may become overly tired.

- Do not leave the trail. Always travel in pairs.
- Avoid heavy packs; packs should be loaded according to the strengths and abilities of the various members of the party.
- Keep a clean camp at all times; this is a must to prevent animals from becoming a problem around the campsite.
- Do not hoard food; it creates interpersonal problems. If food is stored in your tent, pack, or sleeping bag, it is a direct invitation to animal visitors to the campsite.
- Drink plenty of fluids and eat regular meals to keep up your energy.
- Avoid dangerous activities. Do not take any unnecessary risks. Be aware of slide areas and be careful crossing streams.
- Prepare yourself to endure a few hardships; you should not expect to enjoy the comforts of home.
- Carry your personal kit and some first-aid supplies with you at all times. You never know when they will be needed.
- Above all, relax, enjoy nature, and have fun.

In summary, the cardinal rule in hiking is *don't go it alone*. There are too many hazards when hiking by yourself in sparsely traveled areas. These dangers can usually be avoided by selecting a good partner and not straying too far from your group.

Mental Preparedness

It is important to anticipate and prepare for the unexpected. As it is often said, nature is neither friend nor foe, and your survival in the wilderness depends on you and your attitude. One of the most important considerations in surviving a dangerous or life-threatening situation is the ability to overcome fear and panic. Fear may be brought on by a sudden incident such as a bear crashing into your camp, or it may arise more gradually from emotional stress caused by becoming lost or separated from the group. In an uncontrolled situation it can lead to irrational behavior or panic. By recognizing the problem, remaining calm, and using positive thinking, you can condition yourself to control your emotions and avoid panic. Your knowledge, confidence, and self-control will enable you to calmly and methodically work yourself through a potentially difficult situation. The more familiar with and experienced in the outdoors you become, the easier it will be to adjust to emergencies when they occur.

Outdoor and wilderness travelers should anticipate problems and know the steps necessary to solve them. First, and most important, you must be able to recognize the problem. The sooner you realize that it is, indeed, a problem, the easier it will be to solve. Sit down and take the time to logically think out the various alternatives to solving your dilemma. Put aside your promise to return at a certain time or a need to maintain a strict schedule. Develop a plan to solve the problem. As you develop a plan, remember to relate your training experience to the situation. Don't let your fear cause you to forget what you know. Think positively as you carry out this plan. Developing a positive attitude is one of the most important things you can do to overcome fear and work toward a safe survival.

To develop problem-solving skills before going out into the wilderness, place yourself and your group in a hypothetical situation. Decide which are your immediate problems, discuss the seriousness of each problem, and consider possible solutions. Be optimistic in solving the problems, but recognize your weaknesses and limitations. Be sure to utilize the strength and know-how of each member of the group while formulating your plan. An example of developing this problem-solving technique is given in Chapter 22, "Evacuation and Signaling," on evacuating an injured person from the wilderness. This approach can often make a seemingly difficult situation one that can be comfortably managed.

Identifying Some Specific Fears of the Outdoors

Fear may arise very suddenly from the hissing of a rattlesnake or the face-to-face meeting with a large black bear; or it may arise more gradually from the threat of being lost. Loneliness is an inherent fear in the wilderness, especially if one is lost. The possible lack of food, water, and shelter are also fears which confront us in the outdoors or the wilderness. Let us examine some of these concerns in a positive light to lessen anxieties that are commonly associated with them.

Fear of Animals   First of all, you must realize that most wildlife is dangerous if provoked, threatened, or cornered. There is no animal more ferocious than the female badger when you invade her habitat or bother her young. You should give animals the freedom they deserve by avoiding their habitats. Most animals will make every effort to avoid humans; however, some may be attracted by the food that people bring with them. You may cross an animal's path, but few will seek you out. We are, perhaps, most frightened by poisonous snakes, bears, and the great white shark. Knowing and understanding the behavior of such animals can lessen our fear of them while in the outdoors.

Poisonous snakes should be avoided. The most important consideration is where you place your hands and feet, especially on rock ledges and trails where they are often located. Knowing more about their natural habits can prevent injury (see Chapter 9, "Things That Bite and Sting").

The bear is one animal that always seems attracted to campsites because it has a great affinity for refuse and we leave so much of it in accessible places. A bear's curiosity can be discouraged by keeping the camp clear of all food items and refuse. Do not keep any tempting food in the tent or sleeping bags. Thoroughly cleanse all pots and pans after use. If you leave camp, place all food in a stuff sack and secure to a high branch at least 50 yards from the campsite. If a bear enters your camp, make as much noise as possible (yell, bang pans, blow a whistle, etc.) and most important, keep your distance.

Largely because of the movie *Jaws,* much paranoia surrounds the great white shark lurking in our coastal waters. Actual attacks against swimmers are relatively few, but they receive considerable press when they occur. Fortunately, most dangerous sharks (white, blue, thresher, and mako) inhabit the deeper waters off the coast. Occasionally they are sighted along the beaches or near shallow reefs in search of food. It is recommended that you take some precautionary measures in any coastal waters where their presence is suspected.

- If a shark is sighted, get out of the water by swimming directly to shore or climbing back into your boat.
- Divers and snorkel enthusiasts should never swim alone. They should always carry a prod in case the sharks become inquisitive.
- Do not thrash or splash in the water if you suspect that they are in the area. Swim as quietly as possible to get away from them.
- Do not swim in unknown or unclear waters.
- Do not clean fish over the water. The blood and the innards are a direct invitation for dinner.

Fear of Being Lost   Becoming lost or thinking you are lost is one of the greatest concerns that besets an inexperienced person in the wilderness, and it will be intensified by thirst, hunger, cold, and fatigue. The thought of darkness and being alone will also contribute to fear and must be dealt with. While fear is often a normal reaction, many fears are imaginary. Fear can make problems seem more serious than they are, so it is important to control it. Even an experienced woodsman sometimes becomes temporarily lost or confused about present location. With the aid of a good compass and a topographical map (discussed in Chapter 17, "Map and Compass"), which all wilderness travelers should carry, you will be able to establish your bearings. If you are confused about your position or think you may be lost, the first thing to do is *stop*. Find a comfortable place, sit down, and think about your situation. Using your problem-solving techniques, think things out in a realistic manner. If you have only recently strayed from your group, use your whistle to signal your position. Other members of the party probably have discovered your absence already and are concerned with your where-abouts. If there is no response, get out your compass and map and try to determine your exact location and how to get back on the trail. Try to determine where you went wrong or where you missed the trail. If you are still confused, you should *stay put*. For a moment, focus on the beauty around you. You will undoubtedly find a vastness and beauty you have never seen before. Enjoy the peace and tranquillity of the outdoors. When you have rested and cleared your mind, go back to your compass and map. Look for some distinguishing land-marks which correspond to your map in an attempt to gain your bearings. If you are still unsure of your position and it's getting late, think about making camp for the night. *Think positive!* Don't get frustrated! Equipped with your day pack (remember, always carry it with you), you are not in any serious trouble. You can easily provide for yourself for several days or more. You possess skills regarding how to build a shelter, and knowledge of food, water, and signaling, so your problem is not as great as it may seem. Find a good location and build a fire. A fire will cheer you up and provide you with warmth. It will also help combat any fear of the darkness or loneliness which may begin to creep into your mind. The darkness is a common fear. Strange noises, especially at night, are frightening, but usually the fear is unfounded. Eat only a small portion of your rations to ease your hunger. If there is a threat of rain, it is important to provide yourself with an adequate shelter to stay dry. Being refreshed by staying dry, warm, and having something to eat will provide you with a positive outlook toward a safe return.

If you have lost your compass and are confused about your location, allow nature to assist you in establishing your bearing. Look up at the stars at night and find Polaris, referred to as the *North Star*. This star is one of the most important navigational aids available to determine the direction of north. It is the brightest shining star in the northern sky, and stands out among all the rest. It can be spotted by locating the Big and Little Dippers (see Figure 1). The two bottom stars of the Big Dipper will point toward it. Once you have established the direction of north, you can easily find east and west by the position of the sun in the morning. You will observe the sun rising a bit south of east and setting slightly north of west. For example, if you are traveling north, the sun will be at your right in the morning, at your back at high noon, and to your left in the afternoon. Knowing the direction of north will permit you to travel in a relatively straight line during the day.

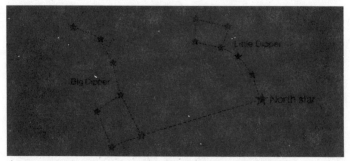

Figure 1 The North Star is an important navigational aid.

Other Methods of Finding Your Way If you still cannot find your way, be alert to any signs of civilization, such as smoke rising in the distance or noises indicating the presence of people. Climb to a higher vantage point so you can obtain a better view and a more accurate direction of the ground. Plot the position with the aid of your map and compass and triangulate the direction you want to travel.

There may be signs of civilization such as a trail or an old logging road. Remember that logging roads will branch off into the woods. If you meet a fork in the road, the chances are that you are traveling in the wrong direction, and deeper into the woods. Turn around and stay on the main road. It is usually the best route to take.

Look for streams or rivers and follow them in accordance with their position on the map. Using the North Star and the sun, you can establish your bearings. Remember that the streams usually flow toward the sea.

If none of these techniques work and you feel hopelessly lost, *don't quit and don't panic.* If you have any woods sense at all (you probably wouldn't be out there if you didn't), you can sustain yourself indefinitely by being knowledgeable in wilderness survival. Meanwhile, find a good spot, stay put, and conserve your energy. Now utilize all the signaling capabilities that you possess to reveal your position. Rescue squads are on duty in most wilderness areas. Once your absence is reported they will soon begin their search to spot your location.

Working in your favor is the strong will to live. If you keep your mind on pleasant things and especially the value of life, you will find the inner strength necessary to survive.

Chapter 17
Map and Compass

People who enter a remote or wilderness area need a good compass and a topographical map of the country in which they intend to travel. Of even greater importance is that they know how to use these two instruments. Wilderness travelers, hunters, and anglers often rely entirely upon another person to get them in and out of the backcountry. Once there, the angler can usually avoid becoming lost by fishing upstream or downstream from the camp. It is not difficult for anglers to establish their present location in relation to the campsite if they stay on the same stream. Hunters or other wilderness travelers are more likely to become separated from the group and lose their bearings. If they cannot establish their position or relocate the trail, they may become lost. Being knowledgeable in the use of the map and compass can prevent this predicament.

Maps

People will often venture into unfamiliar areas without adequate or up-to-date maps. There are numerous maps to select from, but the topographical map is a *must* for the wilderness traveler. Topographical maps are prepared by the U.S. Geological Survey and are the most up-to-date maps available. They are usually made to a scale of 1:24,000 or 1:62,500, which is a simple proportion between the distance on the map and the actual distance on the ground. Topographical maps, called *topos*, are relatively easy to use. The best way to become familiar with their features is to have a knowledgeable person show you how to use them or to enroll in a map-reading course. Topos inform you of changes in elevation within horizontal distances. Compare the various characteristics of the map with the terrain and the features on the terrain. These maps provide a wealth of information about a particular area; they inform you of the topography, the water, the vegetation, and large structures. You will find the topography marked in different tints of brown indicating mountains, hills, valleys, and various contours of the land. Contour lines connect points of equal elevation. If the contour lines are close together, a steep slope is indicated. The water features are marked in blue and indicate bodies of water such as oceans, rivers, lakes, streams, swamps, and marshes. Thin blue lines denote streams, and the heavier lines indicate rivers. The vegetation features marked in green indicate forest or scrub brush. Grassland or barren areas are shown in white. For easier travel it is important to know which land is an open area and which is heavily wooded. The artificial features are marked in black or lavender and indicate roads, trails, railroads, dams, bridges, dwellings, and other structural features.

The topographical map also denotes the magnetic compass declination in degrees, which is explained later in this chapter. Maps are designed so that north is at the top of the map. To your left will be west and to the right is east. You should always read the map by placing it so that the upper part faces north and coincides with the geographic or true north. If the map is properly oriented, all landmarks on the map will line up with the features of the terrain. *Remember to always align the map in this position.* A few additional tips for the use of your map include:

- Study your map carefully; review a small section at a time and visualize the route prior to setting off to walk it.

- Always stop long enough to memorize the major characteristics of the next section of your route.

- Always observe the surroundings (hills, valleys, rivers, prominent landmarks) to see if they match up with the characteristics on the map.

- Occasionally look behind you to identify the area you have just passed. Landmarks will often appear different when viewed from a different direction.

Topographical maps are available from the U.S. Geological Survey (USGS), the National Forest Service, the State Fish and Game Department, and outdoor stores. You can also find maps by checking the Yellow Pages of your telephone directory under Maps. The cost of these maps will range from $1.00 to $2.50. To determine the maps needed for a specific area of the country you should first obtain a map index. These are available from the National Cartographic Information Center, 507 National Center, Reston, VA 22092. Request an index to topographical maps from the U.S. Geological Survey.

When ordering a specific map, specify the appropriate map by name and number. Write to the following addresses to obtain maps of specific areas:

- *East of the Mississippi* The Branch of Distribution, USGS, 1200 East Street, Arlington, VA 22202
- *West of the Mississippi* The Branch of Distribution, USGS, P.O. Box 25286, Federal Center, Denver, CO 80225
- *Alaska* USGS, 520 Illinois Street, Fairbanks, AL 99701
- *Canada* The Map Distribution Office, Department of Mines and Technical Service, Ottawa, Ontario, Canada

The Compass

It is foolhardy to travel into a remote area without a compass. You should select a good compass and learn how to use it. Care must be taken so that it does not become lost or damaged during your outing.

In the selection of the compass you will find a wide variety available, ranging in price from $5.00 to $80.00 and more. There are four basic types of compasses: orienteering, floating dial, cruiser, and fixed dial models. The *orienteering compass* (Figure 1), perhaps the most suitable for the wilderness traveler, has a calibrated collar for setting the angle of declination and is mounted on a rectangular transparent base which makes it a valuable aid in orienting a map. Highly recommended models ranging in price between $6.00 and $30.00 include the Silva Polaris, Type 7NL; the Silva Explorer, Type III; and the Suunto RA-66 Scout. The serious backpacker should consider the Silva Ranger, Type 15TD, or the Suunto RA-69DE Wayfinder.

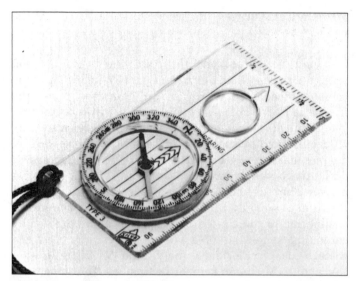

Figure 1 Orienteering Type III Explorer compass. (*Silva Company, Box 966, Binghamton, NY 13902.*)

The *floating dial* compass is one of the easiest to use. This compass is read by simply pointing it toward your objective and reading the degrees directly from the dial, at an index on the compass base. This system is relatively simple as there is nothing to set. The *cruiser compass* is a good instrument for the professional and is similar to a surveyor's compass. It is of high quality and extremely accurate but heavier and more expensive than most. The *fixed dial* is considered for the most part to be inadequate except for the occasional hiker who stays on a well-marked trail. Its use is not recommended. For further information on compasses and compass ratings, refer to the *Backpacking Equipment Buyer's Guide*, by

William Kemsley (see "References and Resources" at the end of this book).

Knowing Your Position In establishing your position with a compass it is important to remember that the compass needle points to an area referred to as the magnetic North Pole. The only time it will reflect a true geographical reading of north is when you are on the line of declination. Usually your position will be several degrees east or west of true north. These degrees or declination values are indicated in all topographical maps. They designate the compass declination within the area covered by the map. The location of the line of declination in the United States can be approximated by extending somewhat of a curved line starting off the eastern coast of Florida, through Lake Michigan (east of Chicago) to Michigan's upper peninsula. To compensate for the angle of declination off this line you must adjust your compass reading by adding or subtracting the declination value from true north. You must adjust your compass in order to utilize your map, which is always oriented to true north. For example, if you are west of Chicago, add the declination value to the compass reading to find true north. If you are east of Chicago, subtract the declination value. You can obtain a declination chart of the United States for 50 cents by writing to the Department of Commerce, Coast and Geodetic Survey, Distribution C44, Washington, DC 20235. Request the Isogonic Chart of the United States, No. 3077.

Guidelines The following guidelines are presented as helpful reminders in the use of the compass:

- Remember, the compass needle points to the magnetic north and not the true north, unless you are standing on the line of declination.

- When you orient the map by using the compass, always place the map on a flat surface, facing true north.

- Always refer to the angle of declination and adjust your compass to coincide with north. The compass declination is often misunderstood or ignored. *Do not disregard its importance!*

- If you do not have a declination chart, you should know the declination angle or variance for your particular locale.

- Always keep metal objects such as knives, axes, flashlights, or belt buckles away from the magnetic needle. They will affect the magnetic needle's true reading.

- Electric power lines and natural deposits of mineral ore will affect compass accuracy.

Triangulation Using a technique referred to as *triangulation,* you can determine your position with the aid of the map and compass. First you need to align your compass to true north with your map facing the same direction. Sight a prominent landmark in the distance and locate it on the map. Take a degree reading on your compass toward this landmark. Draw a line on the map that passes at the same angle directly through the landmark and extend it back to the area you are in. Next sight a second landmark and take another compass reading. Draw a similar line on the map at the appropriate angle and extend it back. The spot where these two lines intersect is your approximate position. If you become familiar with this technique, you will have little difficulty in establishing your position. For example, if you deter-

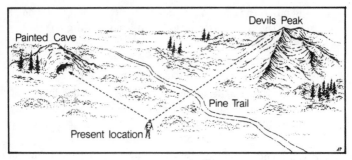

Figure 2 A simple technique to use in determining your position.

mine that you are only a few miles west of Pine Trail, orient your compass and proceed as indicated in Figure 2.

Orienteering Orienteering is a means of finding your way through an area to a preselected destination with the aid of a topographic map and a compass. This is an excellent method of learning basic techniques of map and compass use. Most experts in navigation believe that you can achieve at least the basic understanding of the use of map and compass in a couple of hours. You should start by experimenting with these skills in a lightly wooded area or a city or state park. Through this kind of practice you can gain knowledge of and confidence in their use without the danger of becoming lost. To become proficient in orienteering you must practice these skills many times before embarking into unfamiliar areas. To develop your orienteering skills be sure to read *Be Expert with Map and Compass,* by Bjorn Kjellstrom (see "References and Resources"). For additional information on orienteering write to the United States Orienteering Federation, P.O. Box 1039, Baldwin, MO 63011, or the Canadian Orienteering Federation, 333 River Road, Vanier, Ontario.

Chapter 18
Clothing and Equipment

When selecting clothing and equipment for an outing, prepare to meet the most severe demands of the region in which you plan to travel. Choosing the right clothing will make the trip both comfortable and safe. In meeting your clothing and equipment needs, you should check with a reputable wilderness clothing outlet, especially in the selection of boots, outerwear, and sleeping bags. Most other clothing can be obtained from used clothing stores or army surplus outlets or improvised out of hand-me-downs if large enough and made of the proper materials.

The most important considerations in the selection of outdoor wear are the ability of the clothing to *insulate* the body against the cold, to offer proper *ventilation* in order to keep the person dry, and to provide the maximum *protection* against the severe elements. Observe the following guidelines for purchasing outdoor wear to be used under normal wilderness conditions.

Clothing should not be new and it should be well laundered to avoid chafing. This is a condition often caused by wearing stiff new clothing. In general, cotton is the least irritating material, and synthetic fibers (i.e., rayon, nylon, and orlon) should not be worn next to the skin. If clothing becomes damp from rain, snow, or perspiration, it causes a rapid loss of body heat in a cold environment. In winter areas where the temperature fluctuates, down-filled garments are the best protection against cold, if they do not get wet. Wool is the most ideal clothing for cold-weather travel, as it has the unique characteristic of retaining body heat even if wet. The fibers will wick excessive moisture away from the body to the outer layers to evaporate. This leaves the clothing nearest to the body dry. Virgin wool, lamb's wool, and cashmere cause less itching and provide warmth and ventilation needed in severely cold climates. Thermal underwear, Duofold two-layer underwear, Thermoactyl fiber blend (vinyon and acrylic underwear), and fishnet-weave long johns eliminate the itching caused by wool and have become popular with the hiker in cold climates. The use of several layers of loose, lightweight woolen garments is recommended in order that clothing can be removed or replaced as the demand arises. The layer method of dressing allows air to circulate through the material, removing excess moisture and maintaining body temperature. Properly ventilated rain gear to protect clothing from becoming wet is a must in wilderness travel. A pair of well-insulated waterproof boots with lug soles should be obtained. They should be well broken in prior to travel to prevent blisters. Two pairs of loose-knit socks are recommended: a light undersock and a heavy wool outer sock. In cold climates, two pairs of heavy wool socks are advisable, as the double layer of heavy wool will provide extra warmth.

Head, Face, and Neckwear A hat should always be worn to protect against the sun in hot weather and to retain body heat in cold conditions. A wide-brim felt hat will shed rain; assist in protection of the head, eyes, and ears from the sun; and is ideal for most situations. For the cold, select a cap made of wool or leather fur felt to cover the ears and the back of the neck. Specific arctic face masks are available and should be used in extreme cold, especially in cross-country skiing. Bandanas to protect the neck from the hot sun are advisable, and chin straps are helpful for certain hats to prevent their loss during climbing.

Parka Windbreaker, Rain Gear, and Jackets A lightweight ventile, 60/40 cloth (60 percent cotton, 40 percent nylon) or Gore-Tex parka for wind and rain conditions is recommended. Careful selection of this item should be made for wilderness travel. Probably the best all-around waterproof material available is Gore-Tex. It is a breathing material which lets moisture escape and still keeps out the rain. For thorough waterproofing of this material silicone coating must be applied around the seams. Gore-Tex is expensive but superior to most other rain-and-wind gear.[1] Rain-and-wind pants, worn over the trousers for dryness, are also a necessary item. They should be loose-fitting and have drawstrings around the ankles to keep out the wind, rain, or snow. Gaiters are recommended in snow travel to keep the snow from getting into boots and to help socks and feet stay dry. Down booties are essential in keeping the feet warm or rewarming the

[1] Under extremely damp conditions and for marine wear, Bukflex II may be the material of choice.

feet after a day's hike in the snow. Jackets insulated with down are the most popular due to their lightness and warmth. Another reason for their popularity is that they can also be easily stored in a small pack. They have their disadvantages in outdoor travel, however. If they get wet they are rendered nearly useless, and it is virtually impossible to dry them out in a damp environment. Jackets using polyester (Hollofil II, PolarGuard, and Thinsulate) insulation are somewhat heavier and bulkier than down-insulated jackets and are less expensive. This material can be dried easily in a few hours by shaking or by exposure to the sun and wind. Stuff bags can help keep jackets dry when stored in a backpack. A new vapor-barrier clothing to control the humidity of the body has recently been developed. It essentially retains the body's moisture and slows down its rate of perspiration. Excessive perspiration is vented off through zippered openings.

Shirts, Sweaters, Trousers, and Underclothing A tightly woven woolen shirt is another must for wilderness travel. It should be large enough so that several layers of clothing can be comfortably worn underneath. A good wool shirt can keep a person warm even if wet. Long, loose-fitting sweaters are preferred to allow ample body movement. A tighter weave of the material prevents the loss of body heat and allows adequate ventilation. Lightweight cotton pants or jeans are good for warm weather conditions but loose-fitting woolen pants are best for the cold. Cotton, boxer-type undershorts should be worn by both men and women under normal hiking conditions, especially for the sake of cleanliness.

Boots The boot selected for outdoor travel is most important. It should be sturdy enough to withstand the rigors of the trail and should extend to the ankle for support and protection. Boots too high, rising above the ankle, impair ventilation and freedom of the ankle during climbing. Lugged soles are important to prevent slipping and to provide better support for the foot. They should still be flexible enough for comfortable walking. Boots should fit properly, and it is advised that they be at least one-half size larger and one width wider than the normal street shoe to allow for two pairs of heavy socks. This extra room will give greater comfort through better ventilation, keep the foot drier, and aid in the prevention of blisters. Waterproofing can be improved by treating boots with silicone, or Sno-Seal wax-base boot preservative. Proper drying is essential in the event that they become wet. Different types of boots should be considered for specific types of outings. For example, the lighter, more flexible boot is the best buy for trail hiking. A heavier boot is necessary for the mountaineer.

Gloves and Mittens Lightweight wool, or sometimes cotton, gloves are acceptable in moderate temperatures if they do not get wet. In cold conditions, wool, fiberpile, or fur-lined mittens with nylon waterproof coverings are best to keep the fingers and hands dry and warm. Gloves can be worn inside the mittens so the mittens can be removed to perform certain tasks. It is important to have extra mittens and socks when traveling in a damp, cold environment.

Sleeping Bags and Pads The backpacker should have the lightest bag providing the maximum warmth. Bags should be selected according to the weather and the environment in which a person plans to travel. Essentially, there are two types of sleeping bags, those using down and those using polyester (PolarGuard, Hollofil II, and Fiberfil II) insulation. The primary purpose of the bag is to protect the person from the cold; however, it should offer comfort as well. A sleeping bag should be purchased to fit the individual closely but still offer some freedom for the feet. The general recommendation for sleeping bags is that they be about 2 inches longer and 2 inches larger in girth than your body when you lie in the bag with some clothes on. For cold-weather use, you may desire a slightly larger bag to allow for storage of clothing at the bottom. You should not sleep in the clothing used during the day, as it will have accumulated considerable moisture from perspiration which will cool you down during the night. Down-insulated sleeping bags are light, comfortable, and expensive. It is not advisable to take them on trips in which they may become wet, since you need a dry place to sleep. Insulation from the cold is important in a survival situation. The polyester-insulated bags are slightly heavier and bulkier than down-insulated bags but are very practical for wilderness outings. Extra warmth can be obtained by inserting light flannel linings inside the bag. The new Thinsulate insulation apparently captures the best characteristics of both down-insulated and polyester-insulated products. At this time, however, the sleeping-bag industry has not endorsed its use.

Down versus Polyester Insulation In the selection of a sleeping bag and clothing for a particular trip you need to decide which is the best for your particular needs based upon climatic conditions, cost, and weight. Down-insulated clothing is best in all types of cold, dry conditions; in wind (with adequate wind shell); and in cold, dry snowfall (with minimal physical exertion). Listed below are the advantages and disadvantages of down-insulated clothing and sleeping bags.

Advantages	Disadvantages
Lightweight	No warmth when wet
Very warm	Heavy when wet
Breathable	May require wind shell in high winds
Compressible for storage	
Manufactured in different loft thicknesses for all types of cold conditions	Loss of down if cover fabric is ripped
	Expensive
	Loss of loft when clothing is leaned against, slept on, or sat on

Sleeping bags filled with polyester (PolarGuard, Hollofil II, or Fiberfil II) insulation are the most popular bags made for all kinds of weather. The advantages of this type of bag are these:

- It absorbs less than 5 percent of its weight in moisture.
- It can be easily dried in the sun and wind.
- It retains 95 percent of its loft when wet and retains 65 percent of its insulating capacity, keeping you warm when wet.
- It repels moisture from snow or damp, humid weather.
- It has greater comfort underneath than do down-insulated bags.
- It does not mat, shift, clump, or ball up when wet.
- It is less expensive.

The disadvantages are that they are bulkier and are about 35 percent heavier than down-insulated sleeping bags.

It is no simple task for the average person to purchase a sleeping bag suitable for various occasions. Hopefully this information will help you in your selection.

Foam Pads or Ground Covers Foam pads (or ground covers) are necessary to protect against the dampness and cold of the ground during sleep. An Ensolite closed-cell foam pad ($\frac{1}{2}$ to $\frac{3}{4}$ inch thick) is a good ground cover for the backpacker. It will provide good insulation and protection from the ground with a degree of comfort. The more expensive Duralite and Regalite foam pads are more durable and possess excellent low-temperature characteristics. The best value in foam pads is the Himalayan Industries pad, which is priced at about $8.00.

Packs and Frames Selection of packs and frames should be based upon the nature of the outing. Perhaps the most satisfactory pack for short outings is the aluminum pack frame with one large compartment and pockets on the outside. Short-trip packs do not have the necessary room for equipment during extended travel. The wraparound type, permitting freedom of the arms, is often used in climbing and cross-country skiing. An individual who desires a pack for special purposes for excursions should purchase the kind that will best suit his or her personal needs. The total weight of the pack also must be kept in perspective. Generally speaking, your backpack should not exceed more than 20 percent of your body weight, e.g., 35 pounds for a 175-pound man, 22 pounds for a 110-

pound woman. Younger children's packs should never exceed 16 to 20 pounds.

Tents Tents should be light enough to carry but heavy enough to provide adequate protection against the elements. The more durable the material to withstand the elements of rain, wind, and cold, the greater the weight of the tent. Great care should be taken in selecting tents for extreme cold-weather conditions. The following are essential considerations in the selection and use of tents.

- Choose the proper size of tent based on the number of people using the tent and where the gear is to be stowed.
- Choose the proper-weight tent based on reasonable extremes of weather conditions normally encountered on the trips.
- The floors should be waterproof and contain a minimal number of seams.
- Any floor seams should be waterproofed with a seam sealer.
- Tent sides should be of adequate height to allow occupants to sit up.
- Tent sides should be of a waterproof material several inches above the floor.
- Ventilation at the top and at the opposite ends of the tent is preferable.
- Zippered closures should be simple and sturdy.
- Tents should contain mosquito netting if insects will be encountered.
- A rain fly is mandatory in rain and/or snow conditions and should be free of seams.
- The rain fly should be securely fastened and should not touch the nonwaterproof tent top.

- When selecting the tent site, choose a spot free from sharp objects that might damage the tent floor.
- Tent accessories such as cook holes, snow flaps, snow liners, etc., are usually unnecessary for normal backpacking use.
- A shock cord is invaluable in wind and storm conditions for securing tents.
- The inclusion of 50 feet of nylon cord is vital for emergency conditions.
- Clean mud off the tent and thoroughly dry the tent after each use. Also check seams for leaks and reseal if necessary.

For a complete rating on equipment as to type, quality, and cost, refer to the *Backpacking Equipment Buyer's Guide,* by William Kemsley (see "References and Resources").

Chapter 19

Nutrition: Foraging for Food and Water

Nutrition

Proper meal planning for an extended outing will help make it a pleasurable event. Careful selection of foods can provide satisfying meals and a balanced diet at a reasonable cost. A variety of prepacked items from trail food manufacturers are available in backpacking and outdoor stores. They are well prepared and nutritious but expensive. If you can afford these food products, it is an easy way to travel. Supermarkets and delicatessens have essentially all the same items on their shelves at lower prices, but usually in a heavier form. A substantial savings can be realized by preparing your own foods, and they are usually tastier. Considerations in choosing foods include: weight, packaging, likelihood of spoilage, amount needed, and energy content per unit volume. There are many powdered, dehydrated, vacuum-packed, and freeze-dried products available to the consumer on the grocery store shelf. They include cereal and dairy products, fruits, vegetables, entrees, desserts, trail snacks, and beverages. These foods can be sealed in lightweight, nonperishable containers or plastic freezer bags. It is usually necessary to mix and repackage these items if purchased from the supermarket. Remember to put the mixing directions inside each package.

It is important that the caloric value of each food item be considered while planning the meal. In selecting the foods, a good ratio would be two-thirds carbohydrates (of which 25 percent are sugars), one-sixth proteins, and one-sixth fats. During heavy activity the average adult caloric requirement is increased to approximately 5000 calories daily. On a wilderness outing a person should average between 3500 and 4000 calories for each 2 pounds of food per day. Edwin Drew's *Complete Light-Pack Camping and Trail-Food Cookbook* presents do-it-yourself food preparation and is a must for the wilderness traveler (see "References and Resources"). It emphasizes low-cost foods and established recipes. It also describes the foods offering the best taste, least weight, and highest food value. A popular trail-food item that should be taken on all trips is called *gorp* (trail mix). It provides the body with both quick and long-lasting energy and can be made of a mixture of chocolate chips, candy, raisins, nuts, dried fruit, and granola. The menu should be varied but simple. Mentioned below are a number of basic foods you may consider for the outing. If the trip is only for a few days, fresh fruits and vegetables are always a welcome treat.

Breakfast Pancake, biscuit, muffin, and Bisquick baking mixes. Hot cereals, freeze-dried eggs, bacon, ham, and potatoes. Instant breakfasts and beverages.

Lunch and Trail Snacks Dried meats (beef jerky, beef rolls, meat bars, and pemmican bars), granola bars, cheddar cheese, sunflower seeds, nuts, space bars, cookies, hard candy, dried fruit, bouillon, fruit drinks, and trail mix.

Dinner Soups, main-course entrees, pastas (macaroni, spaghetti, noodles, lasagna), stews, and casseroles. Vegetables, rice, hominy grits, cornmeal, desserts, and beverages.

Beverages Coffee, tea, powdered milk, cocoa, chocolate, fruit drinks, Gatorade thirst quencher, Ovaltine beverage mix, and diet drinks.

Condiments and Miscellaneous Items Flour, sugar, brown sugar, wheat germ, salt, pepper, mustard, cinnamon, powdered cream, syrup, honey, margarine, butter, trail butter, vegetable oils, lard, and bacon grease.

Spices Spruce up dinner mixes with oregano, chives, and sweet basil; and pancake mix with cinnamon and allspice. Other spices: salt, pepper, garlic, curry and chili powders, parsley flakes, dry mustard, and vinegar and oil.

Cheeses Add cheeses to eggs, to onion soup, and to any dinner casserole or lunch menu. Cheeses give extra calories and extra protein.

Foraging for Food

Generally speaking, you should eat only what you can positively identify as edible. The only safe test in eating wild edible foods is to possess knowledge of the plants and flowers in the region in which you travel. The best way to learn about these plants is to travel with someone who can identify and explain their various characteristics. Compare this person's knowledge with a manual on plants. It is advisable to study these manuals before feasting on the wild edibles.

When foraging, do not expend more energy looking for food than the food itself will provide. If your food supply is short, don't waste it. Its nutritional value will aid in maintaining your strength and warmth. Food satisfies hunger and bolsters morale; however, it is not essential for short-term survival. Humans may survive without food for 2 to 3 weeks (except in extremely cold conditions) without any long-lasting adverse effects, provided they have ample water.

Natural foods in the wild are seasonal and abundant in most green areas of the country. The best way to maintain a healthy diet of these foods is to catch fish, dig up roots and tubers, and pick berries. The fish will provide the protein, roots and tubers the carbohydrates, and berries the sugar and vitamins.

Edible plants are often much easier to obtain than animals. Edible parts of plants include the leaves, berries, nuts, tubers, roots, rootstocks, leafstocks, and shoots. The nuts are rich in fats and oils and are usually the most nourishing. Some parts of the plants may be eaten raw, but they usually are easier to digest and more palatable if cooked or toasted over a fire. Boiling is perhaps the best way to cook most edible foods, as it preserves the juices and may remove the tannic acid. Tubers, roots, and rootstocks should be cooked for easier digestion. Pack them in mud or wrap them in foil and cook in the coals of the fire.

To determine whether a plant is edible or not use the "taste test." Place a small amount of the leaf or berry on the tongue. If it is bitter, spit it out. *Do not eat.* If it is not bitter, place a small amount in your mouth, chew it well, and hold it in the mouth for 5 minutes. If there is no bitter taste or burning sensation, swallow it. Wait no less than 4 hours and repeat the test. If there are no ill effects, the plant is generally considered safe to eat. Consider these general guidelines in foraging for food in the wilderness:

- Eating unfamiliar foods may cause serious gastric problems and possible death.

- Animals, birds, and rodents may eat many plants that are highly toxic to humans.

- Avoid plants that have a milky or colored sap (dandelions, milkweed, and wild figs are exceptions).

- *Do not eat mushrooms.* They are usually difficult to identify, highly toxic, and offer little nutrition.

- Avoid dead shellfish or those found in pools with other dead shellfish.

- The nuts or seeds from fruits (cherry, peach, apricot) are poisonous.

- Most blue berries and black berries are edible. Red berries are sometimes edible and white berries should not be eaten.

- The inner bark of many trees (birch, beech, willows, etc.) is edible.

- The nuts from pines and acorns are rich in fats and oils. They should be soaked in fresh water, mulched, and ground into flour.

- Grubs, grasshoppers, and other insects are nutritious and

high in protein. Pull off their heads, boil in water, strain, and you have an excellent broth.

- Animal food is edible and generally more nutritious than plant food. *Do not* eat any of the organs that are lumpy or that contain parasite holes.
- Frogs, lizards, and snakes are edible. Cut off their heads, remove the entrails, skin them, and they are ready for the pot.
- Birds and their unspoiled eggs are edible.
- Snails and clams are edible; cook by boiling or steaming.
- The inside of sea urchins is edible and can be eaten raw.
- *Always drink a lot of water with wild edible foods to ensure better digestion.*

"If you need food, head for the water." The greatest number of edible plants and animals are found near the water. The water, in effect, is your supermarket of the great outdoors.

Table 1 lists common edible plants. It indicates the part of the plant that is edible and the proper method of preparation. Some basic plant terminology will help identify the edible parts.

- *Inner bark* is the thin, watery underlayers of bark located under the outer bark.
- *Leafstock* is the stems that attach the leaves to the plant.
- *Roots* and *rootstock* are knotty spindly fibers that anchor the plant into the ground.
- *Shoots* are the young stems of the plant.
- *Tubers* are the ends of the roots and the underground storage compartment of the plant.

TABLE 1
Edible Plants

Edible Food	Part	Preparation	Edible Food	Part	Preparation
Barrell cactus	Pulp	Raw, boiled	Milkweed	Seed pods, leaves, stalks	Boiled
Basswood	Sap	Drinking	Miners lettuce	Leaves	Raw, boiled
	Buds	Raw, boiled	Mint	Dried leaves	Boil for tea or stew
Beech	Leaves, nuts	Raw, roasted			
	Inner bark	Raw	Nettle	Leaves	Boiled
Birch	Inner bark	Raw	Oaks	Acorns	Grind into flour
Bistort	Flower, stem, root	Raw	Papaw	Fruit	Raw
			Pines	Inner bark	Raw
Blueberry	Berries	Raw		Nuts, seeds	Roasted
Brook saxifrage	Leaves	Raw, cooked	Plantain	Young leaves	Boiled
Bulrush	Young shoot	Raw	Poplar	Inner bark	Raw
	Lower stems	Raw	Prickly pear cactus	Fall fruit	Raw, stewed
Burdock	Roots, leaf, leafstocks	Boiled	Purslane	Leaf, rootstalk	Raw, simmered
Cattail	Roots, stems	Raw	Raspberry and blackberry	Fruits	Raw
	Flower spike	Boiled, roasted	Rose (wild)	Fruits, petals	Raw
Chicory	Seeds	Seasoning	Seaweed	Entire plant	Raw, wash thoroughly
	Leaf, roots	Soups; raw or boiled			

Plant	Parts	Preparation
Chokecherry	Red and black berries	Raw, mash, cooked (remove pits as they contain cyanide)
Clover	Flowers, roots, leaves	Raw
Cranberry	Red and orange berries	Raw
Currant and gooseberry	Berries	Raw
Dandelion	Stem, leaves	Raw, boiled
Dock	Leaves	Raw, boiled
Elderberry	Dried blue or black berries	Raw
Fireweed	Stems, leaves	Boiled
Grasses	Seeds, white tips	Raw
Hazelnut	Nuts	Raw, grind into flour
Hickory	Nuts	Raw
Juniper	Berries	Raw, sun-dried
Lichen	All	Raw, dried, boiled (soak prior to eating)
Maple	Inner bark / Sap	Raw / Drinking
Sedge	Stems, roots	Raw
Serviceberry	Blue berry	Raw, sun-dried
Shooting star	Leaves, stems, flowers, roots	Raw
Sorrel (mountain)	Leaves	Raw, boiled
Spring beauty	Tuber	Raw
Spruce	Inner bark, buds	Raw
Stonecrop	Entire plant	Raw
Sunflower	Seeds	Roast and pound
	Tubors	Raw, boiled, roasted
Thistle (elk)	Young leaf, roots, stalk	Boiled, roasted (peel the stalk)
Watercress	Leaves	Raw, boiled
Water lily	Roots, tubors	Raw, boiled, roasted
Wild onion	Roots, stem	Raw, cooked (knowledge of plant essential)
Willow	Inner bark, shoots, buds	Raw
Yucca	Flowers, buds, flower stalk	Raw, boiled, roasted
Wild strawberry	Fruit	Raw

Note: The leaves of many of these plants are rich in vitamin C if eaten raw. They can be eaten plain or in a salad. Young plants are usually more palatable than old plants.

Water

The basic philosophy on drinking water in the wilderness is *when you are thirsty, drink.* Do not save the water. The minimum daily amount of water needed by the average adult under normal conditions is 2 quarts. In a hot environment or during heavy physical exertion this amount may easily increase to 6 to 8 quarts per day. To carry sufficient water for an outing of several days is impractical due to the weight involved, as 1 gallon of water weighs over 8 pounds.

The water obtained from springs, high mountain streams, and glacial runoff may be safe for drinking. Rainwater that is collected as it falls is considered safe. Fresh snow can be melted and safely used. The rule to be followed when considering drinking any water in the outdoors is: *Water that is near civilization or downstream from any habitation must be considered unsafe unless it is treated.* If you have any doubts about the quality of the water, treat it. The only safe ways to destroy bacteria or other impurities in the water are boiling or chemical treatment. Backpackers and wilderness travelers should be familiar with the various techniques of purifying water.

Boiling   Boiling is the most reliable method of destroying any harmful, infectious bacteria in the water. The water at sea level should be brought to a rolling boil for 10 minutes. It is recommended that the water be boiled an additional 2 minutes for every 1000 feet above sea level to obtain the same results. Chemicals that may be used to purify the water when it is inconvenient to stop and boil it include iodine crystals, iodine drops, Potable Aqua, halazone, and bleach.

Iodine Crystals   The use of iodine crystals is the safest method of purifying water other than boiling. They can be obtained in the standard 1-ounce bottle with a bakelite cap at a local pharmacy. The bottle with the iodine crystals is filled with water and shaken vigorously. Allow the crystals to settle to the bottom of the bottle. When the crystals have settled, pour 5 capfuls of the iodine water solution in each quart of water. *Caution:* Do not allow any of the crystals to spill into the water container. The water container should be shaken and allowed to sit for 20 minutes prior to drinking. If the water is cool, allow it to set for 30 minutes. When the water is cold, cloudy, or suspected of being contaminated, add 7 capfuls of the solution and allow the water to sit for 40 minutes prior to drinking. The water may be flavored with a soft drink mix to eliminate some of the iodine taste. *Remember, the taste of iodine is better than severe stomach cramps and diarrhea caused by impure water.* Iodine crystals will not lose their effectiveness during storage. They may be used for disinfecting water hundreds of times and still retain full strength. *Caution:*

Individuals with a thyroid disorder should not use iodine solutions to purify water.

Iodine Solution   A tincture of 2% iodine is sometimes used to purify water. Five drops are added to each quart of clear water and 10 drops to cloudy water.

Potable Aqua   Potable Aqua is a tablet preparation that contains iodine. When drinking any water that is suspect, add one tablet to a quart of water. Cap the container loosely and allow 3 minutes for the tablet to dissolve. Shake the container vigorously and wait 10 minutes before drinking. If the water is cold, discolored, or dirty it is advisable to use two tablets and wait 20 minutes prior to consumption. These tablets may lose up to one-third of their initial effectiveness when exposed to the air for a period of 4 days.

Halazone (Chlorine Tablets)   Halazone is another widely used water purifying tablet, but it is less effective than Potable Aqua. The tablets will lose their effectiveness if exposed to high temperatures or if exposed to the air. It is recommended that two tablets be used per quart of water and four tablets for cold, cloudy, or contaminated water. Mix the solution as you do Potable Aqua.

Clorox (Bleach)   Clorox may be used to purify water by mixing 1 to 3 drops per quart of clear to cloudy water. After applying the Clorox wait 30 minutes before drinking. *Caution: Do not* use bleach solutions that contain active ingredients other than 5.25% sodium hypochlorite.

Water Usage   Listed below are some general principles regarding water and water usage. They will assist you in determining whether water is fit to drink.

- Water that is cloudy or dirty should be filtered prior to drinking. Water may be filtered through a scarf, wool fabric, sand, or vegetation.
- Free-flowing water is normally safe to drink after purifying.
- Check any stream for obvious contamination. Rivers with habitation upstream are always contaminated and the water needs to be purified.
- Water that contains fish, bugs, and fast-moving insects may be used.
- Beware of any water where there is no movement, algae, or insects in the water. Check for animal tracks around the water.
- Beware of water where dry mineral deposits line the edge. It may indicate an alkaline condition. Alkaline water is not fit to drink.
- Seawater is never safe to drink.
- Do not drink water which runs through poison oak leaves.

Always carry water when you travel. You may survive on a canteen of water daily if you conserve energy and stay out of the hot sun. It may be necessary to ration the water supply but do not save it. A number of guidelines should be considered when you are searching for water. They may not always work, but they bear mentioning.

- Animal trails, the tracks of the animals in the early morning or late evening, usually lead to water. You are usually traveling in the right direction when two trails come together.

- Birds are said to fly away from the water in the early morning and to the water in the late evening. It is worth observing.

- Rainwater can be caught in a tarp or poncho or by other means. Dam up a small gulch to contain the water.

- Snow and ice can be melted. For best results pack the snow prior to melting it.

- Dew that forms on the leaves, grass, or rocks can be sponged and collected.

- The sap from birch, beech, and maple trees can be collected. It also has a high nutritional value.

- Barrel cactus contains a lot of water. Cut off the top and mash the insides with a stick. The pulp of the prickly pear cactus and the fruit of the saguaro cactus contain a great deal of water.

- Topographical maps should be used to locate depressions in the terrain, rivers, lakes, and green areas.

- Look for vegetation. Water may be found in lush, green areas, especially where willows, cottonwoods, bulrushes, and cattails are located. The soil is moist and may necessitate digging down several feet to allow the water to collect.

- Check the sandy areas of the outer banks of dry stream beds, especially near the base of the steep bluffs. It may be necessary to wait several hours for the water to collect after digging the hole.

- In forest areas locate distant streams by the narrow v-shaped drainage cuts between the slopes. Water is often found at the base of these slopes.

- Springs are often located along cliffs in mountainous

areas. Look for the moist areas which are sometimes marked on topographical maps.

- At sea, use a tarp to catch rainwater. Remember, fish contain a water supply.
- Solar stills may be used if you travel in desert areas.

Solar Stills Using a solar still is a simple means of developing your own water supply in an emergency situation. It may produce 1 to 4 pints of water over a 24-hour period. Essentially, the solar still is a large piece of clear plastic draped over a hole. The hole should measure approximately 2 feet in depth and 3 feet in diameter. To collect the water, a canteen is placed inside the hole under the plastic. The plastic is held firmly in position with rocks and sand at the outer edge of the hole. A smooth rock is placed in the center of the plastic to produce an inverted cone-like effect. For best results, the hole should be dug in a moist area and lined with vegetation. A small tube of 5 feet in length is placed in the canteen for siphoning out the water without disturbing the humidity of the still. The components of a solar still (see Figure 1) include:

- Clean piece of 6- by 6-foot plastic (Du Pont's Tedler), rough surface on the inner side.
- Rock or sand holding down the plastic around the edge of the hole.
- Green vegetation lining the hole to create a humid air space.
- Smooth rock placed on the plastic over the center of the hole to hold the plastic in position and produce an inverted

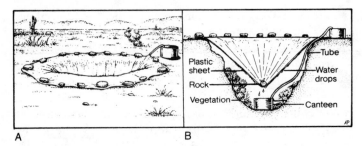

A   B

Figure 1 (a) The solar still will produce water. Practice setting one up prior to using it in a survival situation. (b) A cross-section view of a solar still. Seal edges of plastic with sand to provide greater humidity to the inside area.

cone-like shape from which the water will drip. (Be sure to wrap the rock in a cloth to prevent the rock from becoming hot and burning a hole in the plastic.)

- Canteen or other vessel to collect the moisture which drips down the underside of the plastic.
- Tube to siphon the water from the canteen.

Chapter 20
Predicting the Weather

The ability to predict the weather or forecast an impending storm is vital to anyone venturing into the outdoors.[1] Prior to any outing it is important to obtain information on the climatic conditions of the area you are entering. You should know if the weather fluctuates and what the chances are of rain, wind, cold, or snow. In areas of high elevation and/or where sudden storms are likely to develop, you should be prepared to withstand the rigors of nature. Many a pleasant outing has developed into a frightening experience due to lack of planning. With proper preparation, even the most adverse weather conditions can be withstood. In outdoor travel, bear in mind Benjamin Franklin's often-quoted saying: *"Some are weather-wise, some are otherwise."*

The most dependable method for determining the long-range weather forecast is through the U.S. Weather Bureau. They can usually predict weather conditions with 85 percent accuracy over a 5-day period. Prerecorded

[1] Excerpts from *Weather Wisdom* by Albert Lee. Copyright © 1976 by Albert Lee. Reprinted by permission of Doubleday & Company, New York.

5-day weather forecasts are available by telephoning any of their branch offices. Almanacs, past records, and weather maps are helpful in providing information on climatic conditions in an area. Still, unpredictable atmospheric conditions causing sudden squalls, storms, and whiteouts may quickly develop. An individual who is alert to conditions can make a fairly accurate short-range prognosis on the weather. A number of subtle changes in the environment signal impending weather conditions, and by recognizing these signs a potentially serious emergency can usually be avoided.

Short-Time Warnings In addition to checking the U.S. Weather Bureau forecast you can determine possible changes in the weather by observing the skies, the cloud formations, the wind directions, and the barometric readings. You should also note the habits of the birds, animals, and insects, who are aware of upcoming storms. Many of these signs are part of weather folklore and are surprisingly accurate.

Air Masses There are two types of air masses, warm air and cold air. These air masses do not mix. When they meet, they form high winds, rain, snow, and violent storms. Most violent storms occur when a cold front moves into a warm area, and they give only a short warning. Storms that arise from warm fronts usually can be predicted 1 to 3 days in advance and will usually last longer than those arising from cold fronts.

Cloud Formations One of the best indications that a cold-front storm is developing is a *mackerel* sky. The

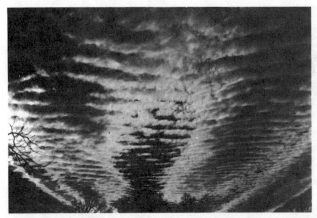

Figure 1 Mackerel clouds (altocumulus); an indicator of a warm-front storm. (*Courtesy of the National Oceanic and Atmospheric Administration.*)

mackerel clouds (altocumulus) appear like herds of little white puffs moving across a clear blue sky (see Figure 1). An old seafarer's adage states, "Mackerel clouds in the sky, expect more wet than dry."

The initial sign of a warm front is the formation of *mare's tails* or cirrus clouds. Mare's tails are long wisps of condensed moisture and are often the earliest sign of a weather change (see Figure 2). If they multiply rapidly, it usually indicates rain or snow in a matter of hours.

Generally, before the warm front can bring on the precipitation (rain or snow) another cloud level will develop called stratus clouds. They arrive in a dull, gray color and are often referred to as a *leaden sky* (see Figures 3, 4, and 5). If this warm front meets with the cold front it will usually bring on a long, steady drizzle. It is said

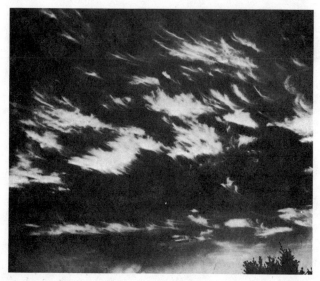

Figure 2 Mare's tail clouds (cirrus); an indicator of a warm front and a sign of a weather change. (*Courtesy of the National Oceanic and Atmospheric Administration.*)

when the mackerel skies meet the mare's tails, it is a sure sign of a violent storm. This means the cold front has moved in on the warm front.

Cumulus clouds are the large billowing ones called *thermal* by meteorologists (see Figures 6 and 7). They develop when a warm air mass rises into the atmosphere. When these clouds are separated, it is usually an indication of good weather. If they continue to grow vertically or if there is a significant increase in number, they are likely to develop into a violent thundercloud. A proverb associated with the cumulus clouds states, "When

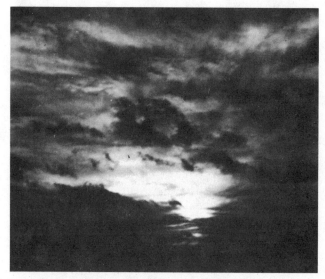

Figure 3 Leaden sky (altostratus clouds). (*Courtesy of the National Oceanic and Atmospheric Administration.*)

clouds appear like rocks and towers, the earth's refreshed with frequent showers."

Whiteouts *Whiteouts,* or the disappearance of terrain under a thick, impenetrable fog or cloud, can completely obscure your mountain trail in minutes. Frequently, a whiteout is so thick that you cannot see your hand at arm's length, let alone trail markers or other landscape features.

To anticipate a whiteout, watch for the rapid formation of a ring of clouds around the very top of the peak

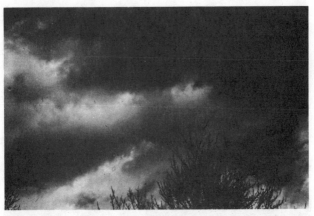

Figure 4 Variation of stratus clouds (nimbostratus). (*Courtesy of the National Oceanic and Atmospheric Administration.*)

above you. It will look as if the peak has speared a few clouds on its tip, although no other clouds are seen anywhere in the sky.

With surprising suddenness, the ring of clouds or cloud "cap" will descend down the mountain slopes, engulfing everything. This phenonemon happens mostly on isolated peaks (Mount Rainier, Mount Shasta, Mount Hood, etc.) which are high in elevation. A whiteout is a hazardous weather condition since it makes further travel treacherous or impossible. Topographic maps, graphs, and trail markers become relatively useless in this weather. In a pinch, you can still rely on sounds (e.g., running water) to act as a guidance system. Making a quick shelter to wait out the whiteout is the best solution.

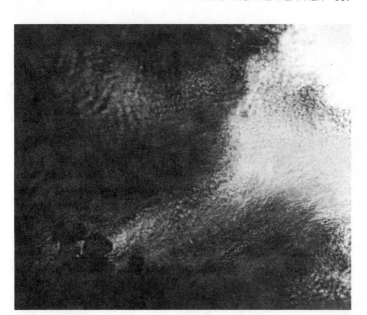

Figure 5 Variation of cirrus clouds (cirrocumulus). (*Courtesy of the National Oceanic and Atmospheric Administration.*)

Wind The wind is a good indicator of ensuing weather conditions. Generally, winds from the north, northwest, and southwest indicate fair weather, while winds from the east, northeast, or south bring rain or snow. Easterly winds often bring some of the severest weather of all. Several old proverbs will help you remember the wind. "Wind in west suits everyone best" and, "A wind in the south has rain in her mouth"; or, "When the wind is from the east, it's fit neither for man nor beast." Remember

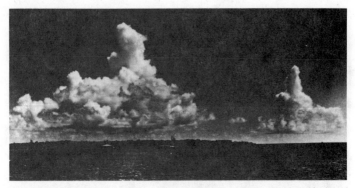

Figure 6 Thermal clouds (cumulus). (*Courtesy of the National Oceanic and Atmospheric Administration.*)

that localized eddies do occur, especially in canyon or mountain areas. Here, simply a reversal of the prevailing wind pattern may indicate the approach of a storm.

Generally speaking, when winds begin to shift about, a storm is brewing. Whirlwinds are considered storm predictors. Veering or backing winds (winds that change directions) indicate change in the weather. "A veering wind will clear the sky, a backing wind says storms are nigh."

Barometer Readings A rising barometer is a sign of good weather, and a falling barometer indicates bad weather ahead. Usually the faster the drop in the barometric pressure, the more severe the weather to come. There are several additional signs for determining barometric lows.

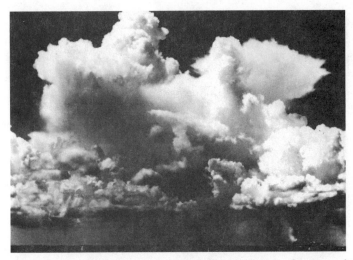

Figure 7 Variation of thermal clouds (cumulonimbus). (*Courtesy of the National Oceanic and Atmospheric Administration.*)

- If smoke rises only a few feet from a fire and tends to level off, it indicates a low barometric pressure with impending rain or snow. If the smoke rises and dissipates quickly, it is a sign of a high barometric pressure and good weather.
- Sounds will carry farther and echoes are more noticeable during low barometric readings.
- Do not disregard the aches and pains of certain individuals in your group. Their bunions or arthritis may give you a clue.

Skies By observing the sky, you can often predict forthcoming weather conditions.

Figure 8 Halo around the sun (cirrostratus clouds). (*Courtesy of the National Oceanic and Atmospheric Administration.*)

- *Corona around the sun* A corona around the sun is often related to a change in the weather. Coronas are small colored rings with red on the outside and blue on the inside. If the corona decreases in size it indicates rain.

- *Halo around the moon* A halo around the moon or the sun is thought to precede rain or snow and generally bad weather. A halo is usually white, much larger than a corona, and does not change in size (see Figure 8). "A large halo round the moon, heavy rains very soon."

- *Color of the sky* Red in the evening sky is considered a sign of good weather ahead, red in the morning, a sign of bad weather. "Red in the morning, sailor take warning, red at night, sailor's delight."

- *Lightning* Red or yellow lightning does not bring rain, while white lightning indicates an upcoming storm. The time between the bolt of lightning and the rumble of thunder reveals your distance from the storm. For example, if it is 15 seconds between, the storm is only 3 miles away (or 5 seconds per mile).

- *Moon* A white-faced moon indicates fair weather, and a red-faced moon says rain is coming. "Red moon doth blow, white moon neither rain nor snow."

Animals, Birds, and Insects Animals, birds, and insects exhibit certain behavior patterns and apparently can anticipate early changes in the weather.

- Deer and elk will usually come down from the high country a day or two before a storm.
- Domesticated animals often appear restless, as is indicated by these sayings: "When a cow tries to scratch its ear, it means a shower is near," or "When the ass begins to bray, be sure we shall have rain that day."
- Chipmunks and squirrels may be busy gathering food.
- If the frogs croak incessantly, it is said rain will soon fall.
- Birds will often perch before a storm. They have difficulty flying in areas of low barometric pressure. They can usually be observed sitting in bunches on limbs, telephone wires, or in the brush. It is stated that "The robin can sense a storm best, it always stays close to the nest."
- Swallows and sparrows are often feeding on low-flying insects that come out when the humidity is high.
- Ants are considered good weather prophets. If the ants are carrying their eggs to the high ground or if you find new earth on an anthill, it is a rain indicator. "Ants that move their eggs and climb, rain is coming any time."
- Spiders will pace actively about their web prior to rain and

desert the web completely when a big rain develops. If you find them weaving their webs, there is good weather ahead. "When spiders weave their webs by noon, fine weather is coming soon."

- Flying insects (mosquitoes, black flies, gnats, etc.) are irritated by the low pressure and high humidity. They are more bizarre in their behavior and bite more fiercely.

- Bees are said to always stay in their hives until after a rain so their wings never get wet.

- Crickets are called "the poor man's thermometer." The exact temperature can be determined by the speed of their chirps. By counting the number of chirps a field cricket makes in 15 seconds and adding the number 37 you will get the exact temperature where they are sitting. If they chirp 50 times in 15 seconds it is 87°F. This method is believed to always render an accurate result.

Numerous other elements of folklore may be used in forecasting the weather. If there is moisture in the air, salt will become damp, and windows and doors may be difficult to open. Flowers are said to stay open all night, stones will sweat, and certain trees will curl their leaves. Perhaps the most dependable sign of all is whether or not there is dew on the grass. Consider these two well-established proverbs: "When the dew is on the grass, the rain will never come to pass," and "When the grass is dry at morning light, look for rain before the night."

No single sign should be used as an absolute indicator of fair weather or an approaching storm. If a number of these signs appear, you can be sure a change in the weather is near. Take notice of the conditions around you. If the sky is gray, the wind is shifting and coming from the south, the smoke hanging in the air, and the robins rattling in the brush, you can be sure a storm is about.

In *Weather Wisdom,* Albert Lee states that there are only two absolute signs for predicting the weather. A temperature rise between 9 and 12 p.m. is always followed by rain, and if you can't see the moon or the stars at night you are probably standing under a cloud. And for all the campers, backpackers, and weekend enthusiasts, "Friday dawn is clear as a bell, rain on Sunday sure as Hell."

Chapter 21
Shelters

One of the most important aspects of survival in the outdoors or wilderness is an adequate shelter. A well-selected tent provides excellent protection against the rain, snow, and insects. However, the proper tent may not always be available in an emergency. This chapter will identify a few simple, easy-to-construct shelters for the wilderness traveler. If you plan to remain in an area for an extended period of time, consider a more elaborate shelter.

The main function of the shelter is to serve your immediate need of protection from the wind, rain, cold, or sun. If you foresee these problems, the general rule is head for the nearest place which affords this protection.

In building a shelter you should consider the protection needed, the length of time it will be used, the availability of material, the time it takes to build, and especially the amount of energy it will take to construct. Usually the more simple the shelter the easier it is to build, thus requiring the least expenditure of energy. Utilize natural windbreaks or available ready-made shelters such as large fallen trees, caves, cliffs, rock ledges, or, possibly, sand dunes. In a forested area it is usually easiest to hollow out a small shelter under a large fallen tree for protection from the wind and rain. This type of shelter can be quickly constructed and will serve your immediate needs until the storm passes.

Caves or overhanging cliffs can be used as emergency shelters when you are traveling in a mountainous area. Caves usually require little preparation to make them habitable. You should always consider that they may have present occupants (e.g., bats, rats, rattlesnakes, or other animals) who call the cave home. Temporary shelters may be provided by a rock ledge, large boulder, or a grove of small trees until the rainstorm passes. With a little ingenuity, emergency shelters can be quickly erected from material such as "space" blankets, a strong, coated-nylon tarp with grommets, or the branches of a tree. Be sure to have plenty of lightweight nylon cord to adequately secure the materials. (If your tarp has no grommets, take a small rock, wrap it in the corner of the tarp and tie it off with cord.)

The bedding for cold-weather shelters can be constructed from evergreen boughs, branches, mulch, or leaves. Make the bed at least 15 to 18 inches thick to insulate adequately from the ground. If boughs are used they should be laid together closely and interwoven with the butt ends toward the feet. This will provide for the greatest comfort and warmth. In hot weather, for relief from the heat of the ground, elevate yourself 6 to 9 inches by lying on piles of clothing, wood, or sleeping bags.

Fires built in an enclosed shelter need proper ventilation. In lean-tos or open-ended shelters a fire may be built at the entrance. Rocks may be used as reflectors if they are placed on the outside perimeter of the fire. You should sleep with your feet toward the fire to receive greater warmth and to permit the warm air to circulate around you, rather than toasting one side or the other.

In selecting the site of the shelter, be alert to some of the hazards that may be incurred by building in the wrong places, for example:

- Where limbs or heavy pinecones may fall from high trees
- Under high trees during a thunderstorm or an electrical storm
- In an area where falling rock, rock slides, or avalanches may occur
- In dry gulches, or creek beds where the streams may rise or flash floods are a hazard
- Under large snow cornices or ledges
- In an area likely to be a bear den or bear run
- In an area infested with ants, mosquitos, or other insects
- In an area where the tide may rise

Lean-to Shelters   A lean-to shelter is used primarily as a windbreak or for protection from the rain. Enclosing the lean-to on three sides provides additional protection and warmth (see Figure 1). Secure a tarp between two trees approximately 5 feet apart. Branches may be placed on the sides to enclose the lean-to on three sides. The structure should face away from the wind.

Downed-Tree Shelter   This is a simple shelter that utilizes the space between the trunk of the downed tree and the ground (see Figure 2). Enlarge the opening on

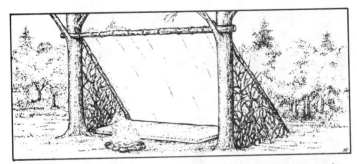

Figure 1 Lean-to shelter; a three-sided lean-to gives greater protection from the wind and rain.

the leeward side of the tree. Branches may be leaned alongside of the trunk to provide additional windbreak. Stretching a tarp or poncho over yourself will provide the essential protection from the rain.

Snow Shelters

Snow is an excellent insulating material and can keep you warm, dry, and safe. A snow cave should be kept simple and small and must have adequate ventilation. The temperature inside the snow cave is maintained by body heat. Body heat plus a lighted candle can raise the temperature inside of a snow cave to approximately 40°F.

Snow-Tree Shelter This shelter can be made by tunneling into a deep snowdrift located at the base of a large evergreen tree (see Figure 3). The tree will provide additional shelter from wind and snow. The snow should

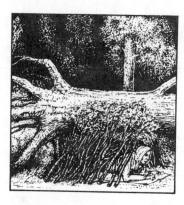

Figure 2 Downed-tree shelter; one of the easiest and quickest shelters to build in providing protection from the wind and rain.

be funneled toward the entrance and placed at a higher elevation than the entrance to provide extra windbreak. The entrance should always be at a slight angle from the wind. For insulation, line the bottom of the shelter with evergreen boughs or a similar material. This shelter will be both dry and protected from the wind.

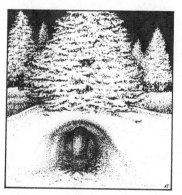

Figure 3 Snow-tree shelter; a quick, easy shelter to build in the snow.

Figure 4 Snow cave; a snow cave will take several hours to build.

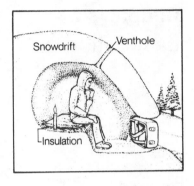

Snow Cave To make a snow cave, it is necessary to dig into a packed snowdrift with a firm crust (see Figure 4). Tunnel upwards at a right angle to the wind. Hollow out an area large enough so that you are comfortable. You should rest on a snow platform a foot or two above the entrance level (it is warmer). Line the cave with boughs for insulation. Several holes should be poked and maintained in the roof for ventilation. The entrance should be made smaller so that it can be partially blocked with packed snow or a similar solid object. Remember, the smaller the shelter the more warmth it will retain.

Shelter building should rate high on your list of survival skills. Taking shelter from inclement weather conditions depends primarily upon your resourcefulness and ingenuity. The best way to save your body in the wilderness is to use your head.

Chapter 22
Evacuation and Signaling

Evacuation

There is no set procedure for evacuating the injured person from a remote setting. Normally the person should be evacuated as soon as it is convenient. The method to be employed depends upon a number of factors: the number, competency, and know-how of the group; the terrain and the degree of difficulty of transportation; the supplies and equipment available; and the distance to communication and/or assistance. Once these assessments have been made, a definite course of action for the rescue can be prescribed.

The general rule prior to evacuating anyone involved in a serious accident is that the victim should not be moved until the initial treatment has been completed. After providing this emergency treatment, make the victim as comfortable as possible. Generally speaking, you should not attempt to move a seriously injured person unless the terrain or weather condition presents a threat to the victim's safety. The overall health and safety of the victim is your prime concern. Often it is more advantageous to move the shelter (tent, sleeping bag, etc.) to the site of the accident. Individuals with non-ambulatory injuries (fracture of the hip, legs, etc.) can be moved after receiving initial care if proper equipment and personnel are available. If the person is ambulatory (able to walk) it is more expedient to assist him or her to camp and tend to the medical condition there.

Note: The evacuation of a seriously injured person from mountainous terrain calls for trained rescue personnel who have the proper equipment to perform such a difficult and often complex task. Search and rescue personnel recommend a minimum of six people to transport a stretcher victim of average size over rugged terrain (see Figure 1). Even then it would be extremely difficult and tiring to move the victim for any extended distance. This type of evacuation may be considered if the injuries are not too serious, the distance is not greater than 3 to 5 miles, adequate personnel and equipment are available, and the victim's spirits are high. Other considerations in evacuating a victim include sending someone for assistance while others care for the victim, waiting with the victim, and signaling for help.

It is necessary to have good leadership qualities to carry out a successful rescue. It is best to select one person to assume this responsibility during the emergency. The leader, with other members of the party, should systematically weigh all the possibilities and determine the best course of action. The leader should be able to calmly delegate responsibility and instruct other members of the party in ways in which they can aid the rescue. He or she should recognize individual expertise in order to achieve the best utilization of the personnel.

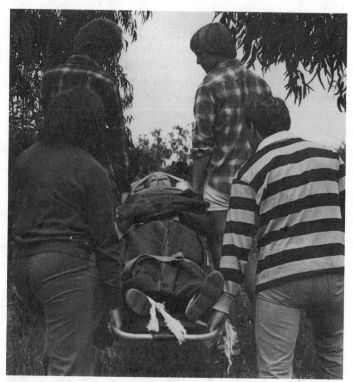

Figure 1 Evacuating the injured requires a minimum of 4 to 6 rescuers over rough terrain. A smaller victim can be adequately transported by 4 rescuers. (*Courtesy of Steve Mitgang.*)

For example, the person with the best background in first aid should stay and tend to the victim. Individuals who are the stronger hikers and most experienced in wilderness travel should be sent for help. The remainder of the group should be kept active in preparing for the rescue. The various tasks could include preparing a shelter; preparing the camp (gathering wood, preparing food, etc.); developing a method of signaling; or preparing a helicopter landing site.

Sending for Assistance   If at all possible, a minimum of two people should be sent to get assistance. A brief written message should be sent with them describing the nature of the accident. This report should include the location of the accident, the condition of the injured, the aid that has been provided, and the method of signaling that will be used. It is important to pinpoint on a map or diagram the exact location of the camp, describe the type of terrain involved, and suggest the method of evacuation deemed necessary. Based upon this information, the rescue team will decide on the method of evacuation. If the accident occurs in a national park, notify the park ranger; if it occurs in any other area, notify the local sheriff's office. *Caution:* Prior to sending anyone for help, wait until weather conditions stabilize. Do not send anyone for help if the weather constitutes a threat to the messenger's personal safety.

Moving an Injured Person   If it is necessary to move an injured person to a more desirable location, do not hurry. No move should be made until a safe plan is developed. A stretcher can be improvised with backpack frames and green sticks cut from small trees. This can be accomplished by lashing and overlapping three backpack frames between two green poles approximately 10 feet in length and 4 inches in diameter. Place the frames across the poles (thicker ends to the rear) and secure them firmly to the poles. The frames can be padded with your Ensolite foam pad, clothing, or a sleeping bag. Firmly strap the victim to the improvised litter prior to any movement. Other methods of transporting an injured person are described in Chapter 15, "Carries and Short-Distance Transfers."

Helicopter Evacuation   A helicopter is usually the preferred method of evacuating a seriously injured person from the wilderness. It reduces the time and the personnel needed and is generally the safest method available. Helicopters can usually land safely at elevations up to 10,000 feet and in winds up to about 35 mph. If the accident occurs at a higher elevation, rescue personnel can bring in the necessary equipment to safely carry out the victim.

A number of considerations should guide the ground party in preparing for a helicopter landing in such a way as to aid the pilot in landing and to protect the people on the ground from possible injury.

- The site selected for the landing should be level and free from any strong wind drafts or surrounding obstructions.
- The direction of the wind can be indicated to the pilot by smoke or cloth streamers tied to low growth. Smoke is usually a good method of indicating the general landing site and the direction and the speed of the wind.
- It is important not to build fires too near the landing site as they would be fanned by the helicopter rotors.
- Individuals on the ground should stay clear of the rotors and wait until they are shut off. If it is necessary for the pilot to hover, be sure to protect the eyes from any flying dirt and stay clear of the rear rotors.

- All individuals should stay clear of the helicopter until the pilot beckons them to approach.
- Assist the rescue crew according to their instructions.

Signaling

Knowing the proper techniques of signaling for help is an essential tool for all people who travel in the wilderness. To be effective, any distress signal, whether visual or aural, needs to be obvious and easy to recognize. The signal must be distinct and literally "stand out" from all other things. The universal signal for help is three of anything repeated at regular intervals. The response to the signal is two distinct sounds or flashes. The signals may include blasts from a whistle, shots from a gun, flares, colored flags, or fire signals. Other methods of signaling include an SOS made by stomping in the snow or using ground lettering made by the placement of rocks. Letters should be made at least 10 feet in size if they are to be effective. Fill in the letters in the SOS with contrasting colors such as green vegetation, dirt, or other objects to make the signal more visible. The standard SOS distress signal can be made by either sound or lights. It is three dots, three dashes, three dots (. . . – – – . . .) repeated at regular intervals. Space blankets which are brightly colored or reflective are also effective signaling devices.

Fires The smoke from a fire can be seen from a considerable distance on a clear day. The three fires should be built in a clearing and in a triangle at least 25 feet apart. Green boughs, grass, or brush will increase the

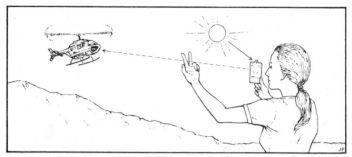

Figure 2 Mirror signaling. The use of the mirror is one of the most effective methods of signaling for help.

white smoke emitted by the fire and make it more noticeable. The use of rubber or plastic will create a dense black smoke. Use dry wood on a fire signal at night so it will burn brightly. If fuel is limited, do not ignite the fire until you hear the rescue plane. Special care must be taken in building fires on a windy day.

Mirror Signals The signal mirror is perhaps the best signaling device of them all (see Figure 2). On a clear day, a signal from a mirror can be seen by a pilot from a distance greater than 10 miles. In using the signal mirror, sight the target through the center hole. Hold the mirror 4 to 6 inches in front of your face and sight through the fingers of the other hand at arm's length. Aim the mirror so the sun spot is reflected slightly ahead of the flight of the plane. If a signal mirror is not available, use any shiny object and wiggle it back and forth to create a visible flash of light.

TABLE 1
Emergency Ground Signals

Signal	Meaning	Signal	Meaning
▬▬▬	= Need a doctor	F	= Need food and water
≡	= Need medical supplies	X	= Unable to proceed
→	= Proceeding in this direction	L	= Need fuel and oil
■	= Need map and compass	LL	= All is well
N–Y	= No or yes	▼	= Safe to land here

Emergency ground signals should be known by the wilderness traveler (see Table 1). These signals should be made in large letters.

Chapter 23

Disasters and Emergencies

Major disasters caused by tornadoes, hurricanes, earthquakes, floods, and blizzards occur in various parts of the country each year. These disasters account for hundreds of deaths, thousands of serious personal injuries, and widespread destruction of property. When such events occur regularly in the same area, people come to expect them. Few people, however, can fully comprehend the impact of these disasters unless they have personally experienced their destructiveness. The unfortunate reality is that most people fail to prepare themselves or their families with safeguards against these life-threatening events.

Certain areas of our country are labeled disaster areas: *tornado alleys* (Midwestern and Southwestern states); the *hurricane coast* (the Gulf states and the Atlantic seaboard); and *earthquake country* (California). There are two important considerations to recognize in all disasters. First, these emergencies will infrequently occur in areas where they are not common or have not previously occurred. For example, in 1979, devastating tornadoes struck areas from Wyoming to Massachusetts, causing many fatalities and widespread damage. People in these communities were unaccustomed to dealing with tornadoes. Second, our travels take us to parts of the country where we know little about conditions indigenous to the area. For example, in August 1978, a late summer tropical storm "blew up" off the Baja Peninsula in California. Flashflooding occurred throughout many of the low desert areas of Arizona and southern California, trapping hundreds of motorists, campers, and vacationers. Snowstorms and whiteouts developed throughout the Sierra Nevada in California. Scores of campers, hikers, and fishermen were totally unprepared for this sudden change in the weather (it had not been predicted in the long-range weather forecast). A number of lives were lost due to hypothermia and exposure to the cold.

Whether you reside in, or travel to, a particular "trouble area" you should prepare yourself and your family for possible emergencies. Being prepared with emergency supplies, knowing the various warning signals, and what to do before, during, and after these events will increase your safety. In preparing for any natural disaster, householders should develop a set of guidelines and equip their homes with the basic necessities for survival. Consider instituting these safety guidelines for your home.

- *Water* Maintain a 2-week supply of water at 7 gallons per person. Remember the extra water that is stored in your water heater and toilet tanks. Have available water purification tablets or Clorox bleach.
- *Food* Maintain a 2-week supply of food. Rely on canned or dehydrated food items. Don't forget the can opener.

- *Utensils*   Have a supply of paper plates, dishes, cups, and other eating utensils available for use.

- *Waste supplies*   Keep a metal waste can with an airtight lid. Have plastic bag liners to enclose human waste.

- *Flashlights*   Have two functional flashlights with extra batteries and bulbs.

- *Matches and candles*   Have a supply of waterproof matches and candles on hand. Exercise caution with the use of these items around possible gas leaks.

- *Utilities*   Know how to shut off the utilities at the main terminals or switches for gas, electricity, and water.

- *Telephone*   Do not use the telephone unless there is an absolute emergency such as a serious injury.

- *Radio*   Have a portable radio as the electricity may be cut off. Know the frequency of the local station broadcasting during emergencies.

- *Family*   Organize a family disaster drill so that each member of the family knows what to do when the disaster occurs.

- *Community*   Know the procedures established for your community disaster programs.

- *Hospital*   Know the locations of your local hospitals and emergency stations.

- *Emergency numbers*   Know and post the emergency numbers of the hospital, fire department, police, sheriff, and ambulance service near all of your phones.

- *Literature*   Obtain specific literature and information on emergencies that may occur in your locale or an area that you plan to visit.

- *First aid*   Maintain an up-to-date first-aid and emergency kit. Enroll in a training program and keep *Common Sense*

Medical Guide with your first-aid and emergency equipment for quick reference.

In addition to the general guidelines suggested for disasters, there are specific actions that should be taken for tornadoes, hurricanes, earthquakes, floods, blizzards, and other emergencies.

Tornadoes Tornadoes are one of the most devastating national disasters in the United States. Tornadoes have been observed worldwide but in the United States are largely concentrated over the Middle West and the Great Plains areas. The National Weather Service refers to storms that contain tornadoes as *outbreaks*. One of the most devasting outbreaks occurred in Xenia, Ohio, on April 3, 1974. A total of 315 people died and damage was in excess of $600 million.

A tornado appears as a violently revolving gray or black funnel cloud and is often referred to as a *twister* (see Figure 1). A tornado appears to blow out in front of a dark, heavy thundercloud, with rain and hail often occurring before and after it passes. The tornado will arise suddenly, giving little advance warning, and pass in a minute or so. Tornadoes usually travel in families (several in an area) from the southwest at speeds of 10 to 50 mph. They are observed at an elevation of 50 to 100 feet above the ground, they average 300 to 400 yards in width, and the family group usually extends less than a mile. Their wind is the strongest produced by nature, and at touchdown it is estimated at 100 to 200 mph and more. Their sound upon approach has been likened to the sound of a million angry bees. They are five times as

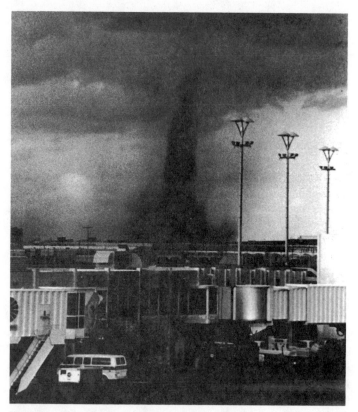

Figure 1 Tornado (Denver Airport, May 18, 1975). (*Courtesy of the National Oceanic and Atmospheric Administration.*)

frequent in the spring and summer months as in winter and fall and may occur at any time of the day or night but are most likely to arise in the late afternoon (4 to 7 p.m.). The powerful winds of a tornado are normally accompanied by tremendous amounts of swirling debris causing widespread destruction of anything in its path. The National Severe Storm Forecast Center states that, since structures and buildings are pummeled so heavily with debris, it makes little difference which side of the house people hide in or whether or not windows and doors are opened in an attempt to equalize the pressure inside the house. The following precautionary measures for tornadoes may lessen any injuries.

Before

- Develop a family preparation plan for tornadoes. Be alert to the fact that tornadoes can occur in your community.
- Keep tuned to your local radio or television station for the latest weather reports. Listen to them carefully.
- If thunderstorms are forecast or observed, watch the sky, especially to the southwest, for a tornado funnel.
- Report any dark, funnel-shaped clouds to the local sheriff's office, police, radio station, U.S. Weather Bureau, or telephone operator.
- Be prepared to take immediate shelter (the best protection is in an underground shelter or cave).
- Shut off electricity and gas if time permits.

During

- In the home, go immediately to a cave, shelter, or basement. Getting under a bench, table, or mattress is preferable to locating in the southwest corner of the house. If at floor level, lie flat on the floor under a heavy bench or table or in a bathroom or closet.
- If outside, go to an open ditch, culvert, gutter, or place of

lower elevation. Do not get under heavy trees or limbs that may topple.

- If in a trailer or mobile home, immediately vacate. Seek shelter in an open ditch or culvert.
- If in an auto, get out of the auto and seek shelter in the nearest ditch or depression.
- In a public building the safest shelter is usually the inside hallway.
- If in school or in a large building, get under the desk or heavy furniture. Avoid windows and heavy objects that may topple. Stay out of gymnasiums or areas that are not well supported.

After

- Do not be curious, stay in the shelter until the tornado passes.
- After the storm, proceed with caution. Be alert to broken glass and fallen power lines.
- Do not light matches around gas lines; use a flashlight that has been switched on away from the hazardous area.
- Check homes for any structural damage: gas and water leaks, electrical problems, and broken sewer pipes.
- Stay tuned to the emergency radio station for information on medical care and emergency procedures.
- Treat any injuries and seek necessary medical help.
- Use your telephone only for emergencies.

Note: Most deaths reported from tornadoes are due to flying debris, falling trees, automobile accidents, and falling power lines.

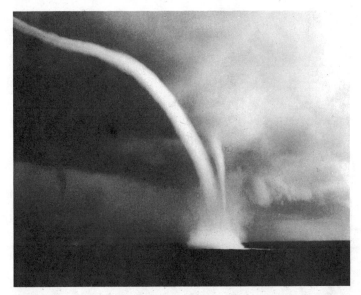

Figure 2 Waterspout (Bermuda, 1961). (*Courtesy of the National Oceanic and Atmospheric Administration.*)

Waterspouts When a tornado appears over a large body of water it is called a *waterspout*. They usually occur between May and October in regions of high temperature. They are caused by unstable air passing over warm water. Waterspouts move at a speed of only 1 to 2 mph but can cause considerable damage to ships, especially small craft. Waterspouts vary in height from 100 feet to a mile or so and appear like giant serpents in the sky (see Figure 2). Hailstones are likely to fall after the waterspout passes.

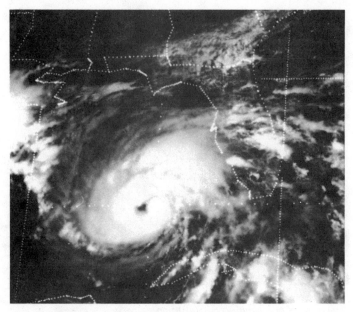

Figure 3 Eye of Hurricane Frederic, September 11, 1979. (*Courtesy of the National Oceanic and Atmospheric Administration.*)

Hurricanes A hurricane is a violent tropical storm. Their destructiveness may be catastrophic. The winds blow counterclockwise around a calm area, called the "eye" of the hurricane (see Figures 3 and 4). They usually occur between July and October along the Gulf States and the Atlantic Seaboard. They develop winds of 125 to 150 mph but tend to weaken and die when the storm moves and remains over land. A hurricane will hit the coastline with heavy rains, often at maximum inten-

U.S. CLOUD COVER
11 SEPTEMBER 1979 1700 GMT
NOAA SATELLITE PHOTOGRAPH
NATIONAL ENVIRONMENTAL SATELLITE SERVICE

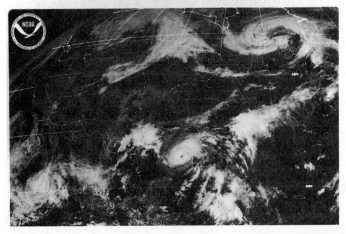

Figure 4 Hurricane satellite (photograph of Hurricane Frederic).
(*Courtesy of the National Oceanic and Atmospheric Administration.*)

sity. The winds and flooding caused by strong tides, often
10 feet above normal, are primarily responsible for its
destructiveness. The average life of a hurricane is about
10 days; however, some have lasted for 3 to 4 weeks and
traveled in excess of 10,000 miles. The eye of the hurricane averages 15 to 40 miles in diameter. In the eye
there is a temporary lull in the movement of the wind
lasting up to a half-hour or more. Remember, if you are
in the eye of the hurricane, the worst part of the storm
often is yet to come. The U.S. Weather Bureau recommendations on hurricanes are listed below.

Before

- Develop a family disaster plan for hurricanes. Obtain information from local authorities.
- Close or board up all windows and shutters.
- Keep your radio or television tuned to the latest U.S. Weather Bureau advice.
- If you are advised to evacuate, do so promptly, travel with care, travel only on the routes recommended. Avoid any low areas as they are prone to flooding.
- If advised to stay, remain indoors, secure all loose objects about the home.
- If advised, shut off the water, gas, and electricity; disconnect electrical appliances.
- If flooding is likely, move furniture to a higher elevation in the house.

During

- Stay tuned to the emergency broadcast station on your car or transistor radio.
- Remain *calm*. Discuss your disaster plan.
- Stay away from large windows, be alert to broken glass or flying debris.
- *Do not be fooled by the calm in the storm.* Do not leave the building as the wind will return, often with increased velocity, from the opposite direction.

After

- Follow the same guidelines advised for tornadoes.
- Do not eat any food that may have been contaminated by the water.

- If an outside well has been flooded, do not drink the water until approval has been granted by health authorities.

Note: Most lives lost in hurricanes are due to automobile accidents, fallen trees, collapsed buildings, and broken power lines.

Earthquakes Many people who reside outside of California and Alaska possess a great fear of earthquakes. An earthquake is a violent shaking of the ground which may last from 5 to 15 seconds or more. Earthquakes in the United States are not as disastrous as most people envision. Geologists assure us that there is no danger that California will fall into the Pacific Ocean. Earthquakes are hazardous but are not as dangerous in terms of fatalities as other disasters. The only two major earthquakes causing large numbers of deaths and severe structural damage since 1951 were the Alaska Earthquake (1964) and the San Fernando Earthquake (1971). The time, place, size, or the probable damage that an earthquake may inflict cannot be predicted. Yet a forecast can be made which points to the possibility of a major earthquake taking place in the United States in our lifetime. This forecast must be put into perspective. We should be prepared, but not paranoid. Earthquakes of various magnitudes have occurred in New England, Virginia, South Carolina, Missouri, Montana, and Hawaii in addition to California and Alaska. These parts of the country remain the most seismically active and earthquake-prone areas in the United States.

Fortunately, we are better prepared for earthquakes in the United States than we were in the past. New building codes have made high-rise buildings safe except for falling objects, plaster, and broken glass. Fires, broken gas mains, and fallen power lines are usually a prime concern. You can reduce earthquake losses in your home by not building on geologic faults, by having insurance, by tying down things that may topple, and by knowing exactly how to react should an earthquake occur. Perhaps the greatest danger of all during a severe earthquake is the reaction of panic. Knowing what to do before, during, and after an earthquake will reduce fear and danger to yourself and others. Given the possibility of a quake, schools should work out safety plans, families should discuss what they need to do, and communities should prepare for the potential dangers.

Before

- Prepare your home against earthquake hazards.
- Provide additional support for water heater and gas heaters. Secure them to the wall with lawn furniture webbing, rope, or wire (see Figure 5).
- Use flexible connections on the gas lines.
- Place heavier objects on lower shelves.
- Anchor top-heavy objects and shelves securely to the wall.
- Secure heavy objects such as bookcases and grandfather clocks to the wall with toggle bolts.
- Avoid hanging heavy mirrors or wall decorations.
- Learn how to turn off the electricity, water, and gas at the main valves.
- Devise safety ledges to support dishes, glasses, and similar objects.

Figure 5 Water heater. Be sure to tie things down that may topple, and use flex hoses on gas and water lines.

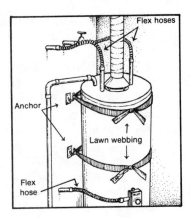

- Maintain flashlights and a battery-operated radio in the home.
- In earthquake areas, support local safety and building codes, especially for schools and community buildings.
- Support programs for a greater awareness of earthquakes and the problems associated with them.
- Have family discussions and develop a safe plan to follow during an earthquake.
- Obtain literature on earthquake safety from the American Red Cross and your local disaster organizations.
- Support research on earthquakes.

During

- First and most important, *stay calm.* Resist the urge to panic. Reassure others and organize your thoughts.
- If indoors, stay clear of windows, mirrors, light fixtures, and other glass objects. Be alert to heavy falling objects

such as a bookcase or a china cabinet. If there is a danger of falling plaster, get under a heavy desk, table, bed, or in a doorway.

- Move to an open space as soon as possible (once the quake stops). *Do not* run outside initially because of the danger of breaking glass and falling objects.

- In a high-rise building, get under a desk. Stay clear of the stairway and of elevators.

- In school, get under the desk. Protect your head and body until the shaking stops. Move to an open space in an orderly manner as soon as the quakes stop. Do not stand near the building. Be alert to broken glass and spilled chemicals.

- In a crowded store, stay calm. Stay clear of nonsecured objects, glass, and decorative ornaments. Exit carefully after the quake.

- If outside, stay clear of buildings and large glass windows to avoid falling glass, brick, and other objects. Avoid broken power lines.

- In an automobile, stop as soon as possible, get out of the car and into an open space. If on or under a bridge, get off or away as soon as possible.

After

- Check and treat any injured person.
- Check all utilities for damage: gas leaks, damaged electrical lines, and broken water and sewage lines.
- Check the building for possible fire hazard, cracked plaster, and structural damage (chimney, too).
- Sweep up any broken glass.
- If the water has been shut off, remember that extra water can be used from the water heater, toilet tanks, or ice cubes.

- Keep tuned to the radio for any damage reports or community instructions. Cooperate fully with public officials and anouncements.
- Be careful in opening closets, storage areas, and china closets as objects are likely to fall out.
- If on a hillside, be alert to landslides, avalanches, and falling rock.
- If on a beach or on the water, be alert to riptides and large waves.
- Be especially alert to the aftershocks. Don't be in too big a hurry to get back into the building. Every earthquake is followed by a number of smaller quakes known as *aftershocks* which are usually of lesser magnitude. (The San Francisco earthquake of 1979 reported a total of 1000 aftershocks during the following 24-hour period.)
- Large earthquakes with their source near the coast may produce a great ocean wave called a *tsunami*. A tsunami is often erroneously reported as a tidal wave.

Note: The reason for the high number of fatalities from earthquakes in many foreign countries is due to the poor construction and location of buildings. Large numbers of deaths occur from collapsed buildings, mudslides, and avalanches which trap people in the debris.

Tsunami If an earthquake occurs along the ocean floor, it may produce a great wave at the ocean's surface called a *tsunami* or a *seismic sea wave*. The most significant tsunami occurring in the United States was generated by the 1964 Alaskan earthquake. At 5 hours and 44 minutes after the quake, the tsunami hit Crescent City, California, with 3- to 6-foot sea waves. The tsunami had been predicted and the townspeople had been evacuated. However, after they returned, there were subsequent waves up to 12 feet at varying intervals which accounted for 11 fatalities. The third to the seventh waves accounted for the most damage to the city. Wait for an "all clear" signal from the authorities before returning to your home.

Floods As a rule, the potential for flooding builds up from heavy rains or melting ice over a period of time. Advance warning of impending flood conditions is usually given to specific communities or locales. Be sure to heed these warnings and follow the advice of the local government. Prompt response to these warnings can ensure your safety and reduce property losses. Follow the same guidelines suggested for tornadoes and hurricanes.

Flash Floods Flash floods commonly occur in foothills, low mountains, and desert areas. If you are traveling in the desert or mountain areas of Arizona, Utah, Nevada, or southern California, anticipate heavy rains during the summer months. If thunderstorms are predicted, be alert to possible flash flooding. If you are intelligently aware of the cloud formation, you can usually predict the impending rains. The cloud formations, especially thunderheads, will build up in early afternoon. Later, at 4 p.m. or so, the skies will darken, wind begin to gust, lightning snap, and thunder rumble, and a torrential rain will follow. Flash floods are common desert hazards during a thunderstorm. They occur very rapidly after the rain begins to fall and can turn a dry creek bed into a raging river in a matter of minutes.

For your personal safety, do not camp in dry creek beds, do not drive into the low desert if thunderstorms are predicted, and do not attempt to cross swollen creeks by foot or auto until the water subsides. Seek shelter and wait out the storm.

Flashflooding may also cause large mud slides in which tons of dirt and debris move down a mountainside. People residing in slide areas should be prepared to evacuate during heavy rains.

Blizzards A blizzard is a severe snowstorm creating drifting snow. Blizzards cause poor visibility and dangerous driving conditions. A blizzard warning is issued by the U.S. Weather Bureau when the winds exceed 35 mph and the temperature drops to 20°F. If a blizzard is forecast, and time permits, go home. If stranded in an automobile, you are presented with a survival situation. Stay with your car unless you can clearly make it to a shelter. Shut off the motor and crack a window to the leeward side for ventilation. If you have planned ahead you will have your emergency supplies of extra clothing and blankets in the trunk (see Appendix D, "First-Aid Kit for the Auto"). You should have added a couple of extra sleeping bags and a shovel to this kit for the winter months. If you periodically run the engine, be sure that the exhaust is clear of any snow. If you are trapped afoot during a blizzard, use the techniques discussed in Chapter 21, "Shelters," to help you survive.

Windstorms Many of our major highways are subject to gusty winds. These winds not only obscure vision with dirt and debris but have the velocity to overturn vehicles. Individuals who drive recreational vehicles or campers or who pull a trailer must be especially alert for these winds. Heed all warnings.

Sand- and Dust Storms   Sand- and dust storms also present hazardous driving conditions. These storms may arise in the desert or an area of arid plowed ground. Listen to your radio for local weather alerts and heed all warnings. If you approach one of these hazards, your best course of action is to turn around, return to the nearest town, and wait it out. If you stop, pull off to the side of the highway and turn on your emergency directional signals. If you are afoot, seek shelter to the leeward side of a large boulder or similar object. Place a bandana over your face and pull your hat down firmly over your head. If you have a blanket, wrap it around you for protection and wait out the storm.

Dust Devil   A common feature of the hot, dry desert is a whirlwind of sand called a *dust devil*. These desert whirlwinds are caused by a high ground-level temperature. If the earth's surface is extremely hot, the overlying air is always affected, causing a turbulence of the air which lifts sand and other debris several hundred feet into the air. The dust devil is short-lived and will pass over in a minute or two. If you are caught in such a disturbance, seek shelter or sit down and protect your eyes and face until it passes. If you are in your auto, follow the same guidelines for a sand- or dust storm.

Fog   Many parts of our country, both coastal and inland, are subject to heavy fog conditions. These fog conditions, especially inland, are referred to as *fogbanks*. They present extremely hazardous driving conditions. Perhaps the greatest danger is that the fogbank will appear suddenly and the driver will be unable to control the vehicle. Be alert to all fog warnings and travel with care. It is not unusual for 10 to 15 vehicles to be involved in a multiple car or truck accident due to a fogbank. If an accident occurs, go back several hundred yards and set out flares. This will warn approaching traffic of the danger ahead.

Lightning Storm Being caught in a severe lightning or electrical storm may be a terrifying experience. Avoid elevated areas as lightning usually strikes the highest object, rebounding from one high object to another until it loses its "zap." If lightning appears, you can usually predict its proximity (see Chapter 20, "Predicting the Weather") and seek shelter in ample time. The danger of being struck by lightning is not great, and if you heed the following basic guidelines you can lessen the danger.

- Seek immediate shelter, especially in a building that has an electrical ground down the side of the structure.
- Get inside your automobile. It provides safety because of its rubber tires.
- If you are in an open field, you may be the best target. Get out of the field or maintain a low profile in a gully or ditch.
- If on a golf course, do not carry your clubs. You have a built-in lightning rod in your hands. The same is true of a gun, fishing rod, or backpack frame. (Get a good distance from anything metal.)
- If you are on a high mountain, get off the top of it. Stay off any exposed slopes. Attempt to find a cave for shelter.
- Stay away from a tall tree or from a single tree regardless of size. There is an added danger of being struck by the falling limbs. (A safe place in the outdoors is in a grove of

trees of the same height, providing that taller trees are in the area.)

- Water is the most dangerous place you can be. Swimmers should immediately leave the water and small boats should get to shore. It is not safe to be above the deck on boats without grounded masts.

- Do not hold hands, and stay a short distance apart from others. More than one person can be struck by the same bolt of lightning.

- If lightning strikes a person, provide BCLS if necessary.

- Treat any wound as a severe burn injury.

Boating Emergencies   All boaters should adhere strictly to the safety rules established by the U.S. Coast Guard on boating. Following these rules will ensure safety for yourself and others. Be sure to provide your boat with lifejackets, flotation devices, and the first-aid and emergency gear indicated in Appendix D, "First-Aid, Emergency, and Specialty Kits." While boating you should follow the same general procedures that you would for any outdoor excursion. File your boating plan indicating your destination, expected time of return, names of the members of the crew, and so forth with the marina office or ranger.

If someone falls overboard, be sure to yell, "person overboard, port [or starboard] side." Toss the person a life ring and maneuver the boat close-by. Shut off the motor prior to bringing the person aboard, to prevent any accident with the propellers. If the boat overturns in rough waters, stay with the boat or wreckage. Do not attempt to swim a long distance to the shore, unless absolutely necessary. Utilize all the flotation devices available. If in a lifeboat, use the signaling techniques explained in Chapter 22, "Evacuation and Signaling." Protect yourself from exposure to the sun as much as possible. *Do not* drink seawater under any circumstances. If you can, catch rainwater with your poncho or clothing.

Airplane Emergencies   When an airplane has to make a forced landing somewhere other than in an open field, a serious accident may occur, resulting in injuries to one or more of the passengers. Your first responsibility is to provide victims with proper medical care. This will be possible if you have equipped your plane with the necessary first-aid and survival equipment indicated in Appendix D. Usually, your best course of action is to stay with the wreckage. It will provide shelter and will be easier to spot from the air. If the plane is not visible, attempt to clear an area where the wreckage can be spotted from the air. Use all the signaling capabilities at your disposal to attract the rescue unit.

Appendixes
Glossary
References and Resources
Index

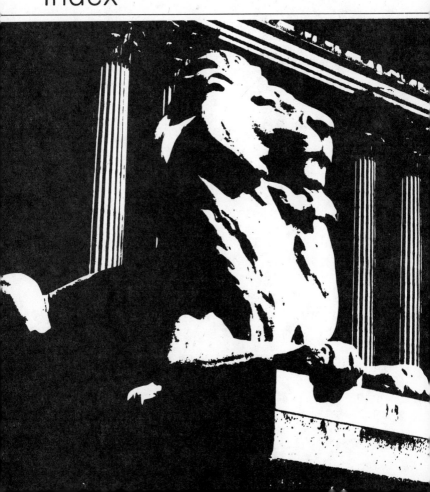

Appendix A
Cancer

The very word *cancer* is often frightening—sometimes too frightening to think about—yet everyone should recognize the possibility of becoming a victim of cancer and be alert to the danger signals. Cancer accounts for over 365,000 deaths annually in the United States. *Early detection is one of the most important measures in the management of cancer.* Cancer can affect any part of the body and spreads rapidly if untreated. The most common types of cancer affect the stomach and the upper respiratory system, the reproductive system (uterus in women and prostate in men), the breast in women, the lungs, the skin, and the blood (leukemia). The American Cancer Society lists seven early warning signals in the prevention of cancer. They spell *caution.*

C hange in bowel or bladder habits

A sore that does not heal

U nusual bleeding or discharge

T hickening or lump in the breasts or elsewhere

I ndigestion or difficulty in swallowing

O bvious change in a wart or a mole

N agging cough or hoarseness

Appendix A is adapted from *Seven Early Warning Signals for Cancer,* American Cancer Society, 777 Third Ave., New York, NY 10017. Used by permission.

If any of these warning signals is present, a physician should be consulted promptly. Individuals can protect themselves by what they *do* or *do not* do. Simple early detection tests will usually reassure a person that he or she does not have cancer. Regular medical examinations are strongly advised. Protective measures against cancer include the following:

- *Do not smoke cigarettes* It is the best way to prevent lung and throat cancer.

- *Do not oversun* If out in the sun a lot, use sunscreens or cover up sensibly. Sunbathe in small doses to prevent skin cancer.

- *Do breast examinations* A monthly examination can help find a breast cancer in time for it to be treated successfully.

- *Do get a Pap test* It is the best way to protect against cervical cancer.

- *Do a guaiac test* This helps detect colorectal cancer early. Your physician can provide you with do-it-yourself slides.

- *Do have an oral exam* Your dentist or physician can easily recognize possible mouth or lymph cancer.

- *Do get a complete checkup* A regular, complete health examination should include a breast exam and Pap test for women, a prostate exam for men, and a proctoscopic exam for everyone over the age of 40.

Cigarette smoking is the *major* preventable cause of cancer. Evidence indicates that moderate to heavy drinking is associated with cancer of the stomach. Cancer of the intestine and the colon may be reduced with diets containing more roughage (raw fruits, vegetables, and whole-grain breads), seafoods, poultry, and less red meat. It is estimated that 75 percent of all cases of Hodgkin's disease (cancer of the lymph glands) could be cured if detected early enough. *Knowing the causes, recognizing the early warning signs, and regular physical examinations are the best guarantees in the prevention of cancer.*

Appendix B
Immunizations and Communicable Diseases

An immunization provides protection against a specific disease. It is not absolute, but it offers a high degree of protection. Inoculations during childhood provide lifetime immunity from only certain viral infections due to the numerous strains of viruses. Specific immunizations are required prior to some foreign travel.

Standard Immunization Recommendations

DPT (Diphtheria–Pertussis–Tetanus) Shots are initially given at 2 to 3 months of age and repeated at 12 months of age and prior to beginning school.

Tetanus Tetanus shots are given in the DPT series, repeated at 18 months of age, and again prior to beginning school. A booster is recommended every 10 years. Obtain a booster for any tetanus-prone wound.

Measles-Rubella-Mumps Measles-rubella-mumps inoculation is given at 15 months of age. Booster shots may be given if child lives in a risk area. *Measles* (red or hard measles) inoculations are seldom given after 15 years of age. *Mumps* shots may be given if not previously inoculated. *Rubella* (German measles) shots are given under certain conditions, but never during pregnancy.

Polio A trivalent vaccine is given at 2 to 3 months of age (three doses at 8-week intervals) and prior to beginning school. A booster may be given prior to foreign travel.

Hepatitis A Immunization may be recommended under certain conditions.

Influenza Immunization is usually given in two injections, 1 to 4 weeks apart. Shots may be given annually for a particular strain of the flu.

Smallpox Vaccinations are no longer given in the United States or required for foreign travel.

Communicable Diseases

If you are planning a trip to certain foreign countries and some areas in the United States, inquire at the U.S. Public Health Department about immunizations against certain diseases. Diseases which require a prophylactic vaccine include those discussed below.

Cholera Cholera is caused by bacteria which are transmitted primarily through contaminated water and uncooked foods. Immunization is required for travelers to certain countries of Asia, Africa, and the Mideast. Booster shots must be obtained every 6 months. The effectiveness of the vaccine is questionable.

Malaria Most malaria cases are seen in the tropics, and the infection occurs through the bite of the infected *Anopheles* mosquito. It can also be acquired through blood transfusions from an infected donor or the use of a common syringe by drug addicts. Prior to travel in malaria-infested areas, consult with a physician for prophylactic treatment. Special protective clothing, mosquito netting, and an insect repellent are necessary. Insect repellent containing Deet (Cutter, Skram, Mosquiton, Off, Repel, or Muskol) is recommended.

Plague Plague is transmitted from rodent to man by the bite of an infected flea, or it may be transmitted from person to person. Isolated cases have recently been reported in the United States. Immunization is recommended for those exposed to plague and people traveling in Southeast Asia. Booster shots are usually obtained every 3 months.

Rocky Mountain Spotted Fever Rocky Mountain spotted fever is caused by the bite or attachment of infected ticks. It is common in areas of North Carolina, Maryland, and Virginia, and in the Rocky Mountain states. Removal of ticks must be immediate to prevent this disease. Inspection of the body at frequent intervals (every 2 to 4 hours) throughout the day to discover tick attachments is recommended. For specific treatment in their removal, see "Tick Bites" in Chapter 9. Individuals who are exposed by travel in infested areas should be vaccinated prophylactically. Protection persists for 6 months, after which time a booster should be obtained.

Typhoid Fever Typhoid fever is caused by bacteria found in water, milk, uncooked food, and vegetables contaminated by sewage. Immunization should be obtained prior to travel to areas where it may be encountered, especially where recent floods have occurred.

Typhus Typhus exists worldwide but is most common in South America and Africa. It is transmitted through the feces of the human body louse. Immunization and louse control are highly effective preventive measures. Kwell is perhaps the most effective medication to eliminate lice from the body. Booster shots are recommended every 6 to 12 months in areas where the disease is prevalent.

Yellow Fever Yellow fever is widespread in parts of South America and Africa and transmitted by the bite of the *Aedes aegypti* mosquito. Immunization should be obtained prior to travel in these areas. Booster shots are given every 10 years.

Appendix C

The Medicine Chest, Guidelines for Safe Use of Prescription Medications, and Vitamins

The Medicine Chest

The Medicine Chest presented here is a list of medications to be considered for common medical ailments on wilderness outings. One medication in each category is usually sufficient. This section is not intended as a self-treatment center or as a substitute for medical advice. The guide does not advocate taking any prescription medication without the specific advice of your physician. For an extended outing your physician may recommend a broadspectrum prescription antibiotic such as tetracycline for infection. *Be alert to side effects.* Some prescription medications including antibiotics are available over the counter in some foreign countries. The use of these medications is not recommended without a physician's advice. Bear in mind that there is no such thing as a completely safe drug. Refer to the next section in this appendix, "Guidelines for Safe Use of Prescription Medications." Explanations for less common abbreviations in the Medicine Chest can be found in Appendix E, "Abbreviations and Symbols."

The Medicine Chest

Ailment	Medication	Adult Dosage	Comment
Allergies	Chlor-Trimeton 4 mg, Allerest, or Benadryl* 50 mg	1 T q4h	Relieves symptoms
Athlete's foot	Tinactin (solution, creams, or powders), Desenex	Apply bid	Tinactin best bet; dry feet and change socks daily
Beestings, wasp, hornet, yellow jackets, fire ants, etc.	Meat tenderizer	1 tsp per teaspoon of water; make paste and apply to area	First remove the stinger and apply ice if available
	Ana-Kit*	Use as directed	For individuals allergic to beestings
Colds	Aspirin	2 T q4h	Take aspirin with food (milk)
	Chlor-Trimeton	1 T q4h	
	Sudafed, Coricidin	1 T qid	
	Neo-Synephrine or Afrin	As directed	Spray nasal decongestants
Cough and sore throat	Robitussin DM, Chloraseptic, Caugh Calmers, or Cepastat lozenges	As directed	Also take saltwater gargles, $\frac{1}{2}$ tsp per glass of water q4h
Constipation	Milk of magnesia	1–2 tbsp at bedtime	For regularity eat plenty of roughage and drink ample fluids
	Fleets Phospho-Soda, Serutan, or Metamucil	As directed	
Diarrhea	Home preparation	As directed	Refer to physician on severe cases (see "Gastroenteritis," Chapter 13)
	Pepto-Bismol or Kaopectate	2 tbsp every 30 min, maximum of 8 doses	
	Lomotil*	1–2 T qid	Not safe for children less than 2 years old

The Medicine Chest (Continued)

Ailment	Medication	Adult Dosage	Comment
HAPE	Diamox* (prophylactic)	As directed by physician in attendance	O$_2$ and descent always best treatment
Headache	Aspirin, Anacin, Tylenol, or Alka-Seltzer Plus	1–2 T q4h	Take with food, milk, etc.
Insect bites	Cutter, Skram, Mosquiton, Off, Repel, or Muskol	Apply liberally to area	For prevention use repellent containing Deet (avoid aerosol cans); for relief, see poison ivy Rx
Itching	Talc Powder, Zea Sorb, or Mexsana medicated powder	Apply to area	Bathe and dry area thoroughly prior to use
	Dermolate, Cortaid	As directed	Contains 0.5% hydrocortisone
	Cornstarch	Soak for 20 min	Mix 1 cup of starch to 4 cups of water and add to warm bath; see poison ivy Rx
Minor cuts, scrapes, and abrasions	Soap and water, Betadine solution, Bacimycin, or similar ointment	Wash thoroughly to cleanse area	Antiseptics may assist in preventing infection
Motion sickness	Marezine or Antivert	As directed	Medication containing meclizine preferred
	Dramamine	1 T 30–60 min prior to departure	
Pain	Aspirin, Anacin, or Tylenol	See headache	
	Aspirin or Tylenol w/ codeine*	1 T q4h	For severe pain

Poisoning (oral)	Syrup of ipecac	1 tbsp w/ ½ glass of water	To induce vomiting repeat in 20 min prn *once only; call physician*
	Activated charcoal	1–2 tsp in 8-oz glass of water	No vomiting indicated; *call physician*
Poison ivy, oak, or sumac	Topsyn Gel*	Apply as directed	Best bet
	Rhuligel, Topic, or Derma Pax		Rhuligel not approved for sumac; cool saltwater compresses relieve itching
	Dermolate, Cortaid	As directed	Contains 0.5% hydrocortisone
Sunburn	Pre-Sun, Pabafilm, Pabanol, or Eclipse	Apply to area prior to exposure	Pre-Sun best bet in sunscreens
	Labiosan	Apply to lips and nose as directed	A glacial cream
	Cortisone Cream*, Carmol HC*	Apply to area	Apply after burns to relieve pain and itching
Toothache	Aspirin or Anacin	2 T qid	
	Oil of cloves	Apply to cavity	Soak in wad of cotton and insert into cavity or to the side of tooth
Upset stomach	Maalox Plus, DiGel, Gelusil M, or Mylanta	Take as directed	Take between meals; chew tablets well before swallowing

* Requires prescription

Guidelines for Safe Use of Prescription Medications

It is important that you thoroughly understand all the instructions on your prescription medication. If you are unsure, ask your physician and/or pharmacist. Listed below are essential guidelines on taking medications.

Do

- *Do* be sure you thoroughly understand all the directions.
- *Do* take only the dosage prescribed by your physician or pharmacist.
- *Do* take the medication exactly as directed (before or after meals, with food or without food, etc.).
- *Do* take the medication on time. (Usually you will have a half-hour leeway, one way or the other.)
- *Do* tell your physician if you are on another medication, either prescription or nonprescription.
- *Do immediately* call your physician if you have any reaction or side effects from the drug that are not expected. (Ask your physician or pharmacist about the side effects that you may expect.)
- *Do* ask your physician any questions you have regarding the drug.

Do Not

- *Do not* take another person's medication.
- *Do not* take any medication after its expiration date.
- *Do not* take medication with alcoholic beverages (check with your physician if there is any question).

- *Do not* try to catch up on your medication if you have missed a dosage.
- *Do not* take more medication than your physician has directed.
- *Do not* take your medication with nonprescription drugs without your physician's advice (some medications will counteract each other).
- *Do not* take medication that produces drowsiness while driving or operating machinery for which mental alertness is necessary.

Remember, any medication in the hands of a child or the wrong person may be dangerous.

Vitamins

A well-balanced diet will normally provide all the vitamins a person needs. Unfortunately many people do not eat a well-balanced diet. One-A-Day multipurpose vitamins with a mineral offer a convenient way to supplement a person's diet, but they are expensive and usually not necessary. They are not a substitute for good, wholesome food. They do not increase pep or resistance to disease. However, taking a normal amount of vitamins prescribed on the bottle is not harmful. What the body does not need usually passes through the system.

Sometimes a vitamin supplement is clearly indicated for a specific deficiency in a person's nutrition. It may be needed during an illness, for a disease, during pregnancy, or after a surgical operation. It should be taken only upon the recommendation of a physician.

Appendix D
First-Aid, Emergency, and Specialty Kits

Both a first-aid and an emergency kit are necessary for the home and travel. The contents of these kits will vary but should include all dressings, medications, and instruments you are likely to need in an emergency situation. The number of items in the kit will depend upon the size of your family or group and the length of trip you have planned. Supplement your emergency kits by making additional bandages from your old, white, lint-free sheets (see Chapter 6, "Dressing and Bandaging Wounds").

For traveling, add some of the items from your family medicine chest, first checking to make sure none of the medications are outdated. Be prepared to encounter some of the frequent vacation ailments which beset the traveler. These include a variety of aches and pains, cold, sore throat, upset stomach, sunburn, insect bite, minor cuts and scratches, constipation, diarrhea, and motion sickness.

First-Aid Kit for the Home

Band-Aid adhesive bandages, assorted
Absorbent cotton
Sterile pads, assorted (1-, 2-, 3-in)
Sterile gauze roller bandage, 2 in
Nonstick pads, assorted (2-, 3-, 4-in)
Bandages, assorted
Butterfly bandages, assorted
Adhesive coverlet bandages
Adhesive tape (1-, 2-in rolls)
Moleskin
Sterile eye pads
Cotton-tip swabs
Elastic bandage, (3-, 4-in)
Rolled cotton bandages (2- to 6-in)
Triangular bandages
Aspirin or Alka-Seltzer
List of emergency numbers

Pocket knife
Oval eye patch
Bar soap
Hydrogen peroxide
Chemical ice pack or ice bag
Chemical hot packs or hot-water bottle
Dual thermometer (oral and rectal)
Large safety pins
Large needle
Large paper clip
Plastic wrap
Tongue depressors
Small flashlight
Small scissors
Rubbing alcohol (isopropyl)
Milk of magnesia
Pepto-Bismol
Poison control kit (syrup of ipecac and activated charcoal)
Common Sense Medical Guide

Note: All personal medications should be kept in a separate area and out of the reach of small children. Any medication that requires a prescription should be used only under the direction of a physician.

First-Aid Kit for the Auto

Include selected items listed under First-Aid Kit for the Home. Additional items should include:

Blankets
Clean sheets and towels
Flares

Large flashlight
Extra rolled bandages
Premade splints

If traveling into remote areas, carry extra water, salt, canned or dehydrated food; extra clothing in a stuff bag; and a ground cloth.

First-Aid Kit for the Boat

Include selected items listed under First-Aid Kit for the Home. Additional items should include:

Extra water
Salt
Canned food
Dehydrated food
Extra dry clothing in a waterproof stuff bag
Blankets

Flares
Fishing equipment (hook, lines, sinkers)
Survival equipment
Waterproof flashlight (extra batteries and bulbs)

Consider items listed under the hiker's Personal Safety, First-Aid, Extended Trip, and Specialty kits, and the Medicine Chest.

First-Aid Kit for the Airplane

Include selected items listed under First-Aid Kit for the Home. Additional items should include:

Canned or dehydrated food
Water
Salt
Clothing
Rain gear

Space blanket
Signal mirror
Survival equipment
Signal flares

Consider items listed under the hiker's Personal Safety, First-Aid, Extended Trip, and Specialty kits, and the Medicine Chest.

FPA Emergency Survival Kit

Basic Equipment

Plastic ground cover
Flashlights
Compass
Pocket knife
Flexible saw
Assorted fish hooks
Gill net

Space blankets
Signal mirror
Waterproof matches
Survival axe
300 ft of 6-lb test nylon line
150 ft of 25- or 30-lb test rope
50 ft of nylon 500-lb test rope

Insect headnet
Whistle
Clothespins
Two-person tube tents

Strobe light
9 ft of surgical tubing
USAF survival manual

Food and Cooking Kit

Stove
Tropical chocolate bars
Foil sheets
Water bag

Variety of soups
Coffee
General food packets

First-Aid Kit

Vitamin tablets
Band-Aid adhesive bandages
Tincture of Merthiolate Sodium
  (antiseptic)
Insect repellent
Unguentine burn remedy
Soap sheets
Kleenex facial tissue

Salt tablets*
Halazone tablets†
Gauze bandage, 2 in
Adhesive tape, 2 in
Sunburn paste
Antibacterial ointment
Bandage compress

* Salt tablets should be crushed and dissolved prior to use.

† Recommend the use of Potable Aqua or iodine crystals for water purification.

Note: The Flying Physician's Association (FPA) recommends an Emergency Survival Kit for airplanes which contains over 60 items. It can be obtained by writing FPA, 801 Green Bay Road, Lake Bluff, IL 60044. The kit is compact in size and weighs 18 pounds.

Kits for the Hiker and Backpacker

The Personal Safety and First-Aid kits for the hiker, backpacker, or outdoors person should contain only the essential items that are most likely to be needed in a wilderness emergency. You should know how to use the entire content of both kits. These kits should be light, compact, and fully stocked. For an extended trip, supplement the kit with additional sterile bandages. It is possible to improvise with most bandages for an emergency. It is recommended that at least one 4-inch elastic bandage be included in the kit. This multipurpose bandage is perhaps the most important single item in the entire pack.

Personal Safety Kit for the Hiker

Plastic water bottle	Compass and map
Signal mirror	Expendable space blanket
Pocket knife	Waterproof matches in water-
Candle	proof case
15 ft of small-size wire	Single-edge razor blade
Flashlight and extra bulb	Fishline (hooks, line, sinkers)
Large safety pins	Assorted Band-Aid adhesive
Sterile pads, assorted	bandages
Elastic bandage, 4-in	Waterproof tape, 1-in width
Granulated salt	Small bar soap
Chap Stick lip balm	Water-purification tablets
Insect repellent	Sunscreen
Snakebite kit	Sunglasses
Pencil stub and small pad	Windbreaker and rain gear
Trail snack, bouillon cubes	Camping permit; fishing and
Phone numbers and several	hunting license
dimes	4 hose champs (hold 2 frame
Whistle	packs to make litter)

Note: A wool stocking cap, wool gloves, and extra socks should be taken in areas of fluctuating weather. Carry all of the above items on your person at all times when you leave the camp. It is of little value to you if it is in your automobile or back at camp when you need it.

First-Aid Kit for the Hiker

Absorbent cotton	Assorted gauze bandages and
Assorted nonstick pads	pads
Butterfly bandages	Gauze roller bandage
Small bar soap	12 in of small rubber tubing
Moleskin	(constricting band)
Aspirin	Tweezers
Meat tenderizer	Needle

Thermometer
Personal prescriptions
Band-Aid adhesive bandages,
  assorted
Elastic bandage, 4-in

Large paper clip
Tincture of benzoin
Waterproof matches (carry in
  both kits)

Supplementary Items

Wire-mesh splint
Antacid tablets
Laxatives
Chemical ice bag
Small pair of scissors
Common Sense Medical Guide

Dextrose, bouillon cubes
Poison ivy–poison oak medication
  tion
Oval eye patch
Antihistamines

Note: Items listed in Personal Safety Kit are not duplicated for the First-Aid Kit.

Specialty Kits

Specialty kits are included below for the day hike, the extended trip, food and cooking preparation, and clothing for winter and summer travel.

Day Hike Kit

Include items listed in the Personal Safety and First-Aid kits. Additional items:

Books (guides to birds, plants)
Bandana
Walking staff
Binoculars
Canteen
Plastic drinking cup
Hat for sun protection

Lunch, bouillon cubes
Appropriate clothing for weather
Small shovel or garden trowel
Magnifying glass
Camera and equipment

Extended Trip or Overnight Trip Kit

Include items listed in the Personal Safety, First-Aid, and Day Hike kits. Additional items:

Pack and frame
Sleeping bag and pad
Moccasins or lightweight shoes
50 ft of nylon cord
25 ft of lightweight wire
Small screwdriver
Safety pins
Hand lotion
Sanitary napkins
Toilet paper
Large spoon
Metal eating bowl or sierra cup

Tent (viseclamps, stakes, rope)
Ground cloth
Repair kit (ripstop tape and sewing kit)
Appropriate clothing for weather
Pliers
Flares
Personal needs (soap, toothbrush, comb)
Razor and blades
Large plastic bag
Hose clamps (4)

Food and Cooking Preparation Kit

The food should be packaged for each meal and each day, and marked in separate plastic bags. Additional items:

Cooking oil
Teflon fluorocarbon-resin coated frying pan
Coffee pot
Collapsible water jug
Extra fuel
Paper towels
Small grill
Funnel
Soap

Condiments (salt, pepper, sugar)
Aluminum cook set or billycans
Plastic soaking bowl with cover
Gas stove with pressure pump
Large spoon
Pot gripper
Scouring pad
Spatula
Channel lock grips
Matches

Clothing for Winter and Summer Travel

Winter Clothing

Inform yourself of the relative merits of wool, down, polyester, and vapor-barrier insulation.

Boots
Knicker socks
Wool pants

Two pairs thin wool liner socks
Two-piece fishnet long underwear

Wool sweaters
Wool cap
Windproof cover
Wool face mask
Insulated bootees
Gaiters
Space blanket
Two pairs wool socks

60/40 parka or windbreaker
Wool mittens
Snow or sun goggles (dark
  glasses)
Windproof pants
Wool felt innersole
Belt or suspenders

Summer Clothing

Boots
Cotton pants
Lightweight shirt (day)
Cotton underwear
Rain suit or poncho
Space blanket
Belt or suspenders

Wool outer socks
Cotton inner socks
Wool shirt (night) windbreaker
Swimsuit
Dark sunglasses

Appendix E
Abbreviations and Symbols

The abbreviations and symbols listed on the facing page
are used essentially as space savers. A number of them
are used in the guide.

AMS	Acute mountain sickness	IM	Intramuscular(ly)
AR	Artificial resuscitation	in	Inch(es)
BCLS	Basic cardiac life support	IV	Intravenous(ly)
		L	Liter
bid	Two times a day	lb	Pound
BM	Bowel movement	max	Maximum
BP	Blood pressure	mg	Milligram(s)
C	Celsius	min	Minute
cal	Calorie	OTC	Over-the-counter (drugs)
CE	Cerebral edema	O_2	Oxygen
CNS	Central nervous system	oz	Ounce
CO	Carbon monoxide	pm	As needed
CO_2	Carbon dioxide	Prog	Prognosis
CPR	Cardiopulmonary resuscitation	pt	Pint
		q4h	Every 4 hours
CVS	Cardiovascular system	qh	Every hour
Diag	Diagnosis	qid	Four times a day
DP	Direct pressure	qt	Quart
DPT	Diphtheria-pertussis-tetanus	RBC	Red blood cells
		RDA	Recommended daily allowance
DSD	Dry, sterile dressing		
DTs	Delirium tremens	Rx	Prescription
ECC	External cardiac compression	S&R	Search and rescue
		sol	Solution
e.g.	For example	SOS	Emergency distress signal
EMS	Emergency medical services		
		T	Tablet(s)
EMT	Emergency medical technician	tbsp	Tablespoon(s)
		tid	Three times a day
etc.	Et cetera (and so forth)	topo	Topographic map
ex.	Example	TPR	Temperature, pulse, and respiration
F	Fahrenheit		
FDA	Food and Drug Administration	TQ	Tourniquet
		tsp	Teaspoon(s)
ft	Foot	V	Victim
g	Gram(s)	WBC	White blood cells
gal	Gallon(s)	wk	Week
GI	Gastrointestinal	w/or c̄	With
h	Hour(s)	s̄	Without
HAPE	High-altitude pulmonary edema	>	More
		<	Less
i.e.	That is	≅	Approximately equal

Glossary

The purpose of the glossary is twofold: to provide brief definitions for medical and wilderness-related terms, and to give a brief description of a number of medical problems not previously identified in the guide.

abdomen The part of the body located between the chest and the pelvis.

acetone breath Odor of the breath of the diabetic person in need of insulin. It is a sweet, fruity odor likened to fingernail polish remover.

acute Being sharp or severe. Having a rapid onset.

airway The tubes or passages which transmit air from the nose or mouth to the lungs.

allergy A reaction of the body tissue to a specific substance. Examples are hay fever, asthma, or hives. Symptoms may be caused by food, heat, cold, dust, animals, feathers, and many other substances.

ammenorrhea The absence or suppression of menstruation.

amnesia The loss of memory; inability to recall past experiences.

anorexia	The loss or lack of appetite.
anoxia	The absence or lack of O_2 in the body cells.
antacid	A substance used to counteract gastric acidity.
antibiotic	A drug such as penicillin commonly used to combat bacteria in the body.
antidote	The substance used to neutralize or counteract the effects of a poison.
antihistamine	A medicine that counteracts the effects of body histamine. Antihistamines are commonly used in the treatment of allergies and other diseases.
antiseptic	An agent that kills or retards the growth of a disease-producing organism.
antitoxin	A substance which is capable of neutralizing a specific toxin (such as tetanus) in the body.
antivenom	An antiserum used to neutralize venom from poisonous snakes, spiders, and other agents.
anxiety	A troubled feeling, a sense of fear or distress.
aorta	The main and largest artery of the body, arising from the heart and supplying the arterial system.
apical	A point of maximum impulse of the heartbeat; generally can be palpated near the left nipple.
apnea	The cessation of breathing.
arrest	A stoppage of breathing (respiration) or of the heart (circulation).
arrythmia	An abnormal rhythm or beating of the heart, often extra beats or skipped beats.
arteriole	A branch of an artery, of a size between the artery and the capillary.

arthritis	An inflammation of the joints of the body. The onset of the disease may be very abrupt and painful.
asphyxia	Suffocation caused by a lack of O_2 or an increase in CO_2.
aspiration	The act of drawing in by suction.
atherosclerosis	Arteriosclerosis or "hardening of the arteries."
athlete's foot	Fungus infection affecting the skin of the feet. The use of a medication such as Tinactin is effective in the treatment.
axilla	The armpit.
axillary temperature	Temperature taken by holding a thermometer under the armpit, close to the body, for approximately 10 minutes.
basic cardiac life support	The administration of cardiopulmonary resuscitation (CPR).
bends	A painful condition experienced by scuba divers, deep-sea divers, and individuals who work in an atmosphere of compressed air, who ascend too rapidly. It causes severe cramps of the abdomen, shoulders, and extremities. Severe pain in the back and joints occurs.
benign	Nonmalignant (not a threat to life).
bland diet	A diet that is soothing in flavor and texture; one that eliminates food causing gastrointestinal irritation.
boils	Acute, tender sores that are inflamed due to bacterial infection. They are usually caused by irritation, friction, excessive perspiration, or clogged pores. They may also develop from a pimple. Special care must be taken with the treatment of boils, especially if they are located in the ear or the nasal pas-

sage. Treat by applying warm compresses frequently to the area. If the boil ruptures, cleanse with soap and water and apply a DSD. Do not squeeze the boil as it may cause spread of the infection.

bolus
A large mass of food that may obstruct the airway.

botulism
A serious type of food poisoning caused by a toxin found in improperly canned food. The toxin cannot be detected by smell or taste. Food boiled for over 20 minutes destroys the toxin.

brachial artery
The main artery of the arm.

bronchitis
An inflammation of the mucous membranes of the bronchial tubes.

café coronary
A condition where a person has incurred a respiratory obstruction due to choking on a large bolus of food. Sometimes mistaken by the nonmedical person as a heart attack.

calorie
A unit of heat; a measurement of the energy value in food.

capillaries
The smallest blood vessels that connect the arterioles and venules.

carcinoma
Cancer.

cardiac
Pertaining to the heart.

cardiovascular
Pertaining to the heart and the blood vessels.

carotid
The main arteries of the neck supplying blood to the brain.

cartilage
A strong elastic connective tissue found in areas such as the ribs and covering the opposing surfaces of movable joints.

catscratch fever
Fever caused by the scratch or bite from an infected domestic cat. The person bitten develops aches, pains, mild fever, and en-

larged lymph nodes in the general area of the wound. Redness and swelling appear at the site of the scratch.

chills
An attack of shivering with a sense of coldness and pallor of the skin. Chills are usually followed by a fever.

chronic
Of long duration.

clammy skin
A damp and usually cool condition of the skin.

clot
A coagulation of the blood.

coma
Unconsciousness.

comatose
Affected with coma.

constricting band
A cravat or other tie used to control external bleeding. It is also used in snakebite injuries.

contact lenses
Small lenses made of plastic or glass that fit directly over the cornea of the eye. If an individual has an infection or an injury of the eye, contact lenses should be removed. Prolonged contact with the lens on the cornea may cause irritation and damage.

contagious disease
A disease that is transmitted directly or indirectly from one person to another.

contaminated
Refers to polluted water, food, or a wound.

contusion
A bruise of the soft tissue of the body. Edema and ecchymosis are present.

crabs
Lice that infest the pubic hairs or other hairs of the body. They itch but do not spread other diseases. They are acquired through person-to-person contact and are successfully treated with Kwell applied as a cream or lotion.

crib death
A sudden and unexpected death of an infant during sleep, usually between the age of 2 weeks and 4 months.

cryotherapy	The use of cold or ice in the treatment of an injury or pathological tissue.
cyanosis	A bluish color of the skin due to the lack of O_2 in the blood. *Cyanotic* is the adjective form.
cyst	A small sac or pouch with a definite wall that usually is filled with fluid. A *wen* is a small cyst of the scalp.
debility	A generally run-down condition.
dehydration	A deficiency in or loss of water from the body.
delirium tremens	Called *DTs,* a symptom complex occasionally resulting from withdrawal of alcohol from the alcoholic. It causes violent shaking, anxieties, restlessness, sweating, depressions, and hallucinations.
demulcent	Fluid or agent used to form a protective coating of the stomach or an agent used to soothe an inflamed or abraded mucous membrane.
dermatitis	An inflammation or state of the skin caused by a number of agents such as poison ivy, poison oak, drugs, and allergic reactions.
diaphragm	The large muscle that separates the chest and the abdominal cavities. Also, a contraceptive device.
dilated pupil	An enlarged pupil of the eye.
diplopia	Double vision.
disinfectant	A chemical that kills bacteria; a germicide.
disoriented	In a state of confusion as to one's surroundings.
distal	Farthest from center or from the trunk of the body.
diuretic	An agent that increases the secretion of the urine from the body.

dyspnea	Difficult or labored breathing.
ecchymosis	A discoloration of the skin caused by blood pooling in the tissue. The color may be bluish initially and later change to a greenish yellow.
eczema	A term applied to rough, red skin which normally appears in patches and which itches. The skin may become swollen or blistered.
edema	A condition in which fluid escapes from the blood vessels into surrounding tissue causing generalized swelling.
electrolyte	The acids, bases, and salts necessary for fluid balance in the body.
expiration	The act of breathing out or expelling air from the lungs (the act of exhaling).
fainting	The temporary loss of consciousness as a result of a decreased blood supply to the brain. Care involves laying the person down on the back and applying a cool compress to the face. Maintain an open airway.
fatigue	A tired feeling, the loss of "pep."
feces	The bowel discharge, stool.
femoral artery	The largest artery of the upper leg.
femur	The thighbone; extends from the knee to the pelvis.
fever	Body temperature above the normal level of 98.6°F.
fibula	The outer and smaller of the two bones of the lower leg.
fracture	Any break in a bone.
gangrene	Tissue death due to obstructed blood supply.
gastrointestinal	Pertaining to the stomach and intestines, abbreviated *GI*.

gingivitis	An inflammation of the gums, characterized by redness, swelling, and bleeding.
gout	A disease marked by acute pain and inflammation of the joints, especially the toe.
groin	The area between the abdomen and the thigh.
hallucination	The act of hearing, seeing, or smelling things that are not present.
hangover	Pain in the head which is caused by over-indulgence in alcoholic beverages. The pain may be dull, sharp, or splitting.
hemophilia	An inherited blood disease in which there is an inability of the blood to clot normally upon injury.
hemorrhoids	Abnormally dilated veins that protrude from the anus; called *piles.* Often bleeding will occur following defecation of a hard stool. Application of warm compresses for 30 minutes four times a day may relieve pain.
hepatitis	An inflammation of the liver.
hiccups	Spasms of the diaphragm, the cause of which is unknown. A common recommended treatment to relieve the hiccups is to eat one teaspoon of ordinary white granulated sugar. If the sugar does not work try a jigger of vinegar.
hoarseness	A condition of the voice resulting from an inflammation or swelling of the vocal cords.
humerus	The bone of the upper arm that extends between the shoulder and elbow.
hypertension	A condition in which an individual's blood pressure is higher than that said to be normal. In general, if the person's systolic pressure is consistently above 140 and the diastolic pressure is over 90, as measured

by a sphygmomanometer, he or she has hypertension. (Normal blood pressure is 100 to 140 for systolic and 60 to 90 for diastolic.) Hypertension is associated with coronary artery disease, strokes, and certain kidney disorders. New drugs have greatly enhanced the physician's ability to manage high blood pressure.

hypoglycemia An unusually low level of sugar in the blood.

hypovolemic An abnormally decreased volume of circulating blood in the body.

hypoxia A state of oxygen deprivation in the body seen, for instance, at high altitude.

ice-water therapy The use of ice water or ice-cold compresses in the treatment of first- and second-degree burns.

immobilization The act of fixing in position or rendering incapable of movement.

inflammation A tissue reaction to an injury or an infection. Pain, heat, redness, and swelling are present.

inspiration The act of moving air into the lungs; referred to as inhalation.

integumentary sheath The skin and its appendages.

intermittent Coming and going at intervals.

-itis Word ending meaning *inflammation*.

jaw-thrust maneuver A procedure used to open the airway, especially if a neck injury is suspected. The jaw is lifted and pulled forward to prevent the tongue from blocking the airway.

jet lag A physical state that occurs following a long airplane flight over several or more time zones. Tiredness, decreased mental acuity, and discomfort are common symptoms.

Several hours of sleep immediately after the flight will aid in alleviating this condition.

kidneys Organs located in the abdomen that filter the blood, regulate the salt and water content of the body, and excrete the urine.

laryngectomy The surgical removal of the larynx (voice box), usually because of cancer.

laryngitis An inflammation of the larynx causing dryness and hoarseness.

laxative A drug used to promote bowel movement, as in the alleviation of constipation. Do not give laxatives in the presence of severe abdominal pain.

ligament A fibrous tissue that connects bone to bone or bone to cartilage. It supports and strengthens the joint.

litter A stretcher (a *Stokes litter* is a basket stretcher).

liver A large organ located in the upper right side of the abdomen. It serves many functions and is essential for life.

lockjaw An early symptom of tetanus characterized by spasm of the muscles of the jaw (see "Tetanus" in Chapter 13).

malaise A generalized feeling of bodily discomfort and fatigue.

malignant Cancerous.

mandible The bone of the lower jaw.

melancholia A mental depression often characterized by marked apathy.

migraine A specific type of a headache, usually severe. It may be preceded by visual disturbances and accompanied by nausea.

mole A discolored spot that may or may not be

elevated above the skin's surface. It is usually harmless unless irritated. Any enlargement or change in the mole should be seen by a physician.

mononucleosis
An acute viral infection, commonly called *mono,* prevalent in young adults. It is often accompanied by a sore throat, headache, fever, fatigue, chills, and a general run-down feeling.

motion sickness
Nausea, dizziness, and perhaps vomiting, caused by motion while traveling in a boat, plane, or car. It may be minimized by taking a medication such as Meclizine or Dramamine 30 to 60 minutes prior to departure.

mucus
A sticky, viscid fluid secreted by the mucous membranes which line the nose, stomach, urinary tract, and other hollow organs of the body. Mucus from the bronchial tubes of the lungs is referred to as *phlegm.*

nausea
A sensation of discomfort in the region of the stomach, often with a desire to vomit.

necrosis
Tissue death due to cellular damage.

otitis
An inflammation of the inner, outer, or middle ear.

oxygenated blood
Blood that is combined with oxygen.

palate
The roof of the mouth and the softer curtain separating the mouth from the throat.

pallor
Paleness of the skin.

palpate
To examine the body by feeling with the hands and fingers.

palpitation
An abnormally rapid heartbeat.

paraplegia
A paralysis of the lower portion of the body.

paramedic
A trained medical assistant who participates in rescue operations.

patella	The kneecap.
pediculosis	A skin disease due to infestation by lice.
pelvis	The basinlike cavity in the lower part of the trunk.
pharyngitis	An acute inflammation of the throat.
pimples	Small prominent inflamed elevations of the skin associated with infected sebaceous "oil" glands.
pleural cavity	The space between the parietal and visceral layers of the pleura around the lungs.
precordial	Pertaining to the area overlying the heart.
prone	Lying in a flat position, face down.
prophylactic	Taking measures in the prevention of a disease.
psittacosis	A viral disease, found in certain birds, called *parrot fever.* It is highly contagious to humans and produces atypical pneumonia.
psoriasis	A chronic skin disease characterized by large, red, scaly patches.
pulmonary	Pertaining to the lungs.
pulse	A rhythmical throbbing (recurrent wave of distention) of an artery in response to contractions of the heart. The normal pulse rate in adults is 60 to 90 beats per minute; in children and infants it is 100 to 120 beats per minute.
pus	The fluid that accumulates usually centrally in an area of inflammation. It is generally yellow to greenish in color.
quadrant	One of four sections of the abdomen divided for descriptive or diagnostic purposes, i.e., right upper, left lower.
radius	The outer, shorter bone of the forearm.

rale	An abnormal fine, wet, crackling sound that is heard in the chest upon either inspiration or expiration.
rash	A general term identifying an eruption or "breaking out" of the skin. A reddish coloration in the skin which may be caused by an infection or an irritation. It is present in diseases such as measles and scarlet fever.
regurgitation	The return of fluids or solids to the mouth from the stomach. *The act of vomiting, upchucking, or barfing.*
respiration	The exchange of O_2 and CO_2 in the tissues of the body (the act of breathing).
resuscitation	The procedure used to revive, or attempt to revive, someone whose heart function and/or respiration has failed.
rigidity	Stiffness or tenseness. Inability to bend.
rigor	A sudden chill with a high temperature causing trembling. Also applied to a state of stiffness in a muscle.
rose fever	Hay fever attributed to inhaling rose pollen.
roughage	Materials in certain fruits, vegetables, and cereals which are not completely digested by the intestine. Plenty of water or fluid should accompany the consumption of roughage.
rump	The buttocks.
rupture	A tear or break of any tissue or organ.
salmonella	A bacteria acquired by eating contaminated food such as poultry, eggs, dairy products, fish, and uncooked vegetables.
salt solution	A solution of salt and water (saline solution).
sarcoma	A tumor, often highly malignant.
scab	The crust of a sore, ulcer, or wound.

scabies   A highly communicable skin disease caused by a mite.

scapula   The shoulder blade.

sedative   An agent that exerts a calming effect or quiets nervous tension and induces sleep.

seizure   A sudden attack, a pain, or more commonly, a convulsion.

semiconscious   Partially conscious.

semirecumbent   In a reclining but not fully lying down position.

shin   The portion of the leg between the ankle and knee; the front edge of the tibia.

shingles   A viral infection of the nerves. It is usually mild in children and most common after the age of 50. Chills and fever may accompany small blisters that develop at the site of the infected nerve.

shin splints   A term used to describe a pain medial to the Achilles tendon or along the tendon, or a pain of the medial aspect of the anterior tibia. For treatment, see "Tendonitis" in Chapter 7.

shivering   The shakes or trembling caused by chills, fever, or fear.

signs   Features that can be observed, e.g., watery diarrhea, dilated pupils, pallor, etc.

sore   A tender or painful lesion of the skin.

sphincter   A muscle that encircles a duct, a vessel, or an opening. It can contract and constrict the opening.

sphygmoman-   An instrument used to measure arterial
ometer   blood pressure.

spineboard	A wooden board used to evacuate a victim who has a suspected spinal injury.
spleen	An organ lying in the upper left side of the abdomen.
sterile	Being free of all germs or living microorganisms (aseptic).
sternum	The breastbone.
stupor	A state of diminished sensibility.
subclavian artery	The large artery at the base of the neck, supplying blood to the arm.
subcutaneous	Beneath the skin.
sunstroke	An illness caused by prolonged exposure to the sun (see "Heatstroke" in Chapter 11).
supine	Lying on the back, face upward.
swimmer's ear	An infection of the ear canal often caused by failure to completely dry the ear canal after swimming.
syncope	Fainting or swooning; a loss of blood flow to the brain causing temporary unconsciousness.
symptoms	Features of an illness of which the person complains, e.g., pain, nausea, etc.
tachycardia	A very rapid heartbeat and corresponding fast pulse of over 100 beats per minute.
Tel-Med	A telephone system employing 3- to 5-minute tape-recorded messages on medical, dental, and health care information.
temperature, body	The degree of heat of the body. The normal temperature is 98.6°F if taken by an oral thermometer under the tongue. It is 99.6°F if taken rectally, and 97.6°F if taken in the axilla. Body temperatures below 95°F and above 106°F indicate a serious medical condition.

temporal	The region of the forehead, relating to the temples.
tendon	A fibrous cord which attaches muscle to bone.
therapy	Treatment of an injury, disease, or pathological condition.
thready	A pulse lacking fullness; thin and feeble.
tibia	The larger of the two bones of the lower leg (the shinbone).
tonsillitis	An inflammation of the tonsils in the back of the throat, usually due to a strep or viral infection. Common signs include fever, headache, sore throat, and pain on swallowing.
toothache	Pain that may be caused by an infected tooth; an obvious cavity may be present. A sharp pain, chills, slight fever, and a sensitivity of the involved tooth are present. Inserting a cotton wad soaked in oil of cloves into the cavity is often recommended to relieve pain. See a dentist as soon as possible. A temporary filling can be made from zinc oxide powder and eugenol. Check with your dentist for details.
tourniquet	A constricting device such as a cravat bandage used to control bleeding from an extremity if all other measures fail. Do not use unless absolutely necessary.
tracheotomy	A surgical opening of the trachea (windpipe) to create an airway. It is a last-resort measure to relieve an obstructed airway.
traction	The act of pulling or stretching a part. It often refers to a method of setting a broken bone and the application of a splint.
trauma	An injury or wound.

tremor Involuntary trembling (quivering or shaking).

trichinosis A disease contracted from eating raw, undercooked, or unprocessed pork or pork products infected by the roundworm *Trichinella spiralis.* If the pork is thoroughly cooked until brown at the center, the parasite (roundworm) will be destroyed.

trunk The body with the exception of the head and the extremities (the torso).

tularemia An infectious disease associated with handling or eating infected wild rabbit. It also may be contracted by drinking infected water, handling infected birds, or through contact with infected ticks or the deer fly (also called rabbit or deer fly fever). Preventative measures include wearing gloves and a long-sleeved shirt while handling or preparing these animals, cooking the food thoroughly, boiling drinking water, and carefully removing ticks.

tumor A swelling or an enlargement of tissue. It may or may not be malignant.

ulcer An open sore or lesion of the skin, often accompanied by the formation of pus; an erosion of the mucous membrane such as the stomach or duodenum.

ulna The inner and larger bone of the forearm.

unconsciousness The state of being insensible; not conscious.

uremia A toxic condition associated with the failure of the kidneys.

vaccination An inoculation with a vaccine to establish resistance to specific diseases.

vapor-barrier system A type of clothing that allows the release of excessive perspiration. It includes a net undershirt, a vapor-barrier shirt, and a polyester jacket. The shirt and the jacket vent perspiration through underarm zippers.

vascular system	The system that distributes the blood throughout the body. The heart, blood vessels, lymphatics, and their parts.
venom	Poison injected by some animals and insects.
ventilation	The act or process of breathing, the inspiration and the expiration of air from the lungs. Also, the airing of a closed space.
venule	A small vein that connects the capillary with the vein.
vertebrae	Any of 33 bony segments of the spinal column. There are 7 cervical, 12 thoracic, 5 lumbar, 5 sacral, and 4 coccygeal vertebrae that comprise the spinal column.
virus	A class of small organisms that cause a variety of diseases.
vital signs	Signs observed in order to determine the physical state of the individual. They include the pulse, blood pressure, respiratory rate, skin color, and level of consciousness.
vomitus	The fluid or substance that is expelled from the stomach through the mouth.
warts	Growths on the skin, usually appearing on the hands, feet, and face. If they are bothersome or become enlarged they should be seen by a physician.
wheal	An irregular, raised, blanched area of the skin, surrounded by redness, often produced by a sting, an injection, or an allergy.
wheezing	Difficulty in breathing producing whistling sounds, commonly occurring in respiratory ailments such as asthma or croup.
windpipe	The air passage from the larynx to the lungs.
xiphoid process	The cartilage at the lowest portion of the sternum. The tip of the sternum.

References and Resources

References

An extensive listing of reference material is presented for those who desire more information on a specific area. The books marked with the asterisks I have found especially valuable in one way or another.

Aaron, James, E., et al.: *First Aid Emergency Care, Prevention and Protection of Injuries,* 2d ed., Macmillan, New York, 1979.

*Accerano, Anthony J.: *The Outdoorsman's Emergency Manual,* Stoeger, South Hackensack, N.J., 1977.

*American Academy of Orthopaedic Surgeons, Committee on Allied Health: *Emergency Care and Transportation of the Sick and Injured,* 2d ed., Banta, Menasha, Wis., 1977.

American Heart Association: "Standards for Cardiopulmonary Resuscitation (CPR) and Emergency Cardiac Care (ECC)," in *A Manual for Instructors of Basic Life Support,* Dallas, September 1977, revised 1980.

American National Red Cross: *Advanced First Aid and Emergency Care,* 10th ed. rev., Doubleday, Garden City, N.Y., 1973.

————: *First Aid and Personal Safety,* 2d ed., Doubleday, Garden City, N.Y., 1979.

Angier, Bradford: *Feasting Free on Wild Edibles,* Stackpole, Harrisburg, Pa., 1972.

Baake, Thomas: "Wilderness Medicine, a Matter of Survival," *The Physician and Sportsmedicine,* vol. 6, no. 11, November 1978, pp. 133–144.

Battan, Louis J.: *The Nature of Violent Storms,* Anchor Books, Doubleday, Garden City, N.Y., 1961.

Berglund, Berndt: *Wilderness Survival,* Scribner, New York, 1974.

*Berkow, Robert, M.D. (ed.): *The Merck Manual of Diagnosis and Therapy,* 13th ed., Merck, Rahway, N.J., 1977.

Blosser, John, M.D.: "Wilderness Medicine," *Emergency Medicine,* vol. 7, no. 6, June 1975, pp. 22–43.

Brennan, William T., and D. Ludwig: *A Guide to Problems and Practices in First Aid and Emergency Care,* 3d ed., Brown, Dubuque, Iowa, 1976.

Breyfogle, Newell D.: *Techniques of Cardiopulmonary Resuscitation for Rescue Personnel,* rev. ed., University of California Press, Santa Barbara, Calif., 1978.

Bridge, Raymond: *High Peaks and Clear Roads, a Safe and Easy Guide to Outdoor Skills,* Prentice-Hall, Englewood Cliffs, N.J., 1978.

Brack, Richard, M.D.: *The New Handbook of Prescription Drugs,* rev. ed., Ballantine Books, New York, 1975.

Brown, Terry, and Robert Hunger: *The Concise Book of Outdoor First Aid,* Vanguard, Ellenburg, Wash., 1978.

Burt, Calvin, and R. Dawson: *Wilderness Pocket'n' Pack Library,* Life Support Technology, Manning, Oreg., 1974.

*Chatton, Milton J., M.D.: *Handbook of Medical Treatment,* 5th ed., Jones Medical, Greenbrae, Calif. 1977.

*Clark, Charlotte B.: *Edible and Useful Plants of California,* University of California Press, Berkeley, 1978.

*Cohen, Irving (ed.): "Jaws That Bite, Things That Sting," *Emergency Medicine,* vol. 10, no. 7, July 1978, pp. 24–59.

Cole, Warren H., and Charles Puestow: *Emergency Care, Surgical and Medical,* 7th ed., Appleton-Century-Crofts, New York, 1972.

Consumer Reports Editors: *The Medicine Show,* Pantheon, New York, 1974.

Cooley, D. J., (ed.): *Better Homes and Gardens Family Medical Guide,* rev. ed., Better Homes and Gardens Books, Meredith, Des Moines, Iowa, 1978.

Diamond, Don (ed.): *Poisonous Plants of Southern California,* County of Los Angeles, Department of Arboreta and Botanic Gardens, Arcadia, Calif.

Dreisbach, Robert H., M.D.: *Handbook of Poisoning,* 9th ed., Lange Medical, Los Altos, Calif., 1977.

*Drew, Edwin P.: *The Complete Light-Pack Camping and Trail-Food Cookbook,* McGraw-Hill, New York, 1977.

Eastman, Peter F., M.D.: *Advanced First Aid for All Outdoors,* Cornell Maritime, Centerville, Md., 1976.

Fear, Gene: *Surviving the Unexpected Wilderness Emergency,* rev. ed., Survival Education Association, Tacoma, Wash., 1975.

Ferber, Peggy (ed.): *Mountaineering: Freedom of the Hills,* 3d ed., Fail-Ballou, Bingham, N.Y., 1974.

Forgey, William W., M.D.: *Wilderness Medicine,* Indiana Camp Supply Books, Pittsboro, Ind., 1979.

Fosnot, Hal (ed.): "Responding to the Poison Call," *Patient Care,* December 15, 1978, pp. 98–149.

*Graedon, Joe: *The People's Pharmacy,* Avon Books, Hearst, New York, 1977.

Grant, Harvey, and Robert Murray: *Emergency Care,* Robert J. Brady, Prentice-Hall, Bowie, Md., 1971.

Green, Martin: *A Sigh of Relief: The First Aid Handbook for Childhood Emergencies,* Bantam, New York, 1977.

Greenback, Anthony: *A Handbook for Emergencies,* Doubleday, Garden City, N.Y., 1975.

Hafen, Brent, and Keith Karren: *First Aid and Emergency Care Workbook,* Morton, Denver, 1980.

Hafen, Brent, and Brenda Peterson: *First Aid for Health Emergencies,* West, New York, 1977.

Hart, John: *Walking Softly in the Wilderness,* Sierra Club Books, San Francisco, 1977.

Heimlich, Henry J., M.D.: "The Heimlich Maneuver: Where It Stands Today," *Emergency Medicine,* vol. 10, July 1978, pp. 89–101.

*Henderson, John, M.D.: *Emergency Medical Guide,* 4th ed., McGraw-Hill, New York, 1978.

Hobler, P. G. H. (ed.): "Venomous and Poisonous Marine Animals," *Practice of Medicine,* vol. 9, 1975, pp. 1–23.

Jelenki, Carl, M.D.: "Emergency Treatment of Small Burns," *Hospital Medicine,* vol. 2, no. 1, January 1975, pp. 92–96.

Johnson, Loren A., M.D.: *Survival Manual,* Alpine Aid, Ventura, Calif., 1973.

*Kemsley, William: *Backpacking Equipment Buyer's Guide,* Collier Books, Macmillian, New York, 1978.

*Kjellstrom, Bjorn: *Be Expert with Map and Compass: The Orienteering Handbook,* rev. ed., Scribner, New York, 1976.

Kodet, E. Russell, M.D., and Bradford Angier: *Being Your Own Wilderness Doctor,* Stackpole, Harrisburg, Pa., 1978.

Kornbluth, Alfred W.: *First Aid for Boaters,* Crown, New York, 1979.

*Lee, Albert: *Weather Wisdom,* Dolphin Books, Doubleday, Garden City, N.Y., 1977.

Mitchell, Dick: *Mountaineering First Aid,* 3d ed., Snohomish, Snohomish, Wash., 1977.

Moriarty, Richard W., M.D.: "In Case of Poisoning," *Drug Therapy,* vol. 9, no. 8, August 1979, pp. 101–103.

Nelson, Dick, and Sharon Nelson: *Desert Survival,* 2d ed., Tecolote, Glenwood, N.Mex., 1978.

Nourse, Alan E., M.D.: *The Outdoorsman's Medical Guide,* Harper & Row, New York, 1974.

Olson, Larry Dean: *Outdoor Survival Skills,* Pocket Books, Simon & Schuster, New York, 1976.

Parcel, Guy S.: *First Aid in Emergency Care,* Mosby, St. Louis, Mo., 1977.

*Petzoldt, Paul: *The Wilderness Handbook,* Norton, New York, 1974.

Plorde, James J., M.D.: "Current Management of Infectious Diarrhea," *Drug Therapy,* vol. 9, no. 8, August 1979, pp. 41–54.

Powledge, Fred: *Backpackers Budget Food Book, How to Select and Prepare Your Provisions from Supermarket Shelves with Over 50 Trail-Tested Recipes,* McKay, New York, 1977.

Rothenberg, Robert E., M.D.: *The New American Medical Dictionary and Health Manual,* rev. ed., Crown, New York, 1975.

*Russell, Finlay E., M.D.: *Snake Venom Poisoning,* Lippincott, Philadelphia, 1980.

Rustrum, Calvin: *The Wilderness Route Finder,* Collier Books, Macmillian, New York, 1978.

Russell, Finlay E., M.D. et al.: "Bites of Spiders and Other Arthropods," *Current Therapy,* H. F. Conn, M.D. (ed.), Saunders, Philadelphia, 1974, pp. 865–867.

Saunders, Charles F.: *Edible and Useful Plants in the United States and Canada,* Peter Smith, Magnolia, Mass., 1976.

Schifferes, Justus: *The Family Medical Encyclopedia,* rev. ed., Pocket Books, Simon & Schuster, New York, 1976.

Snyder, Donald R. et al.: *Handbook for Emergency Medical Personnel,* McGraw-Hill, New York, 1977.

"Standards and Guidelines for Cardiopulmonary Resuscitation (CPR) and Emergency Cardiac Care (ECC)," *Journal of the American Medical Association,* vol. 244, no. 5, Aug. 1, 1980, pp. 453–509.

Steele, Peter, M.D.: *Medical Care for Mountain Climbers,* William Heinemann Medical Books, London, 1976.

The Tacoma Mountain Rescue Unit: *Outdoor Living, Problems, Solutions, Guidelines,* P.O. Box 696, Tacoma, WA 98401.

Thomas, Clayton, M.D. (ed.): *Taber's Cyclopedic Medical Dictionary,* 12th ed., Davis, Philadelphia, 1973.

Thomas, Dian: *Roughing It Easy,* Brigham Young University Press, Provo, Utah, 1974.

Thomas, Lowell J., and Joy Sanderson: *First Aid for Backpackers and Campers,* Holt, New York, 1978.

Thompson, Steven, and Mary Thompson: *Wild Food Plants of the Sierra,* Wilderness Press, Berkeley, 1972.

Tucker, J. V., and M. Kimball: *Poisonous Plants in the Garden* University of California Agricultural Extension Service, AXT-22, Berkeley, 1966.

U.S. Department of Defense, Federal Emergency Management Agency: *In Time of Emergency,* rev. ed., U.S. Government Printing Office, Washington, 1976.

Watt, Michael, M.D.: *Mountain Medicine,* Van Nostrand Reinhold, New York, 1976.

Watt, Norman, F.: *Instant Weather Forecasting,* Dodd, Mead, New York, 1968.

Weeden, Norman F., *A Survival Handbook to Sierra Flora,* Interface California Corporation at Graphic Arts Center, Portland, Oreg., 1975.

*Wilkerson, James, M.D. (ed.): *Medicine for Mountaineering,* 2d ed., Mountaineers, Seattle, 1975.

Wingert, Willis A., M.D., and Jack Wainschell, M.D.: "A Quick Handbook on Snake Bites," *Medical Times,* vol. 105, no. 4, April 1977, pp. 68–75.

Resources

First-Aid, Outdoor, and Wilderness Suppliers This section provides a listing of outdoor specialty stores, first-aid equipment suppliers, and commercial trail food products. Free catalogs are available from most of these outlets.

Alpine Aid, *Specialty First Aid and Survival Kits for the Great Outdoors,* 141 North Ventura Avenue, Ventura, CA 93001.

Backpacker Books, *The Wilderness Bookstore,* Main Street, Orwell, VT 05760.

Backpacker's Pantry, Dri-Lite Foods, Incorporated, 8607 Canoga Avenue, Canoga Park, CA 91304.

Don Gleason's Campers Supply, Inc., 33 Pearl Street, North Hampton, MA 01060.

Dyna-Med, *Emergency Care Products, First Aid and Rescue Equipment,* 6200 Yarrow Drive, Carlsbad, CA 92008; tel. (800) 854-2706; California only: (800) 542-6012.

Early Winters Ltd., 110 Prefontaine Place South, Seattle, WA 98104.

Eastern Mountain Sports, Incorporated, Vose Farm Road, Peterborough, NH 03458.

Forest Mountaineering, 1517 Platte Street, Denver, CO 80202.

Granite Stairway Mountaineering, 3040 State Street, Santa Barbara, CA 93105.

Great Pacific Iron Works, P.O. Box 150, Ventura, CA 93001.

Indiana Camp Supply Company, P.O. Box 344, Pittsboro, IN 46167.

L. L. Bean, Incorporated, Freeport, ME 04033.

Mountain House, Oregon Freeze Dry Foods, Incorporated, P.O. Box 1048, Albany, OR 97321.

Mountainaire Foods, 4206-H Sorrento Valley Boulevard, San Diego, CA 92121.

Mountain Safety Research, Incorporated, 631 South 96th Street, Seattle, WA 98106.

Natural Food Backpack Dinners, P.O. Box 532, Corvallis, OR 97330.

Northwest River Supplies, P.O. Box 9243, Moscow, ID 83843.

Orienteering Services USA, P.O. Box 1604, Binghamton, NY 13902.

Paul Petzholdt, Wilderness Equipment, Lander, WY 82520.

Recreation Equipment, Incorporated, P.O. Box C-88125, Seattle, WA 98118.

Rich-Moor Products, Rich-Moor Corporation, P.O. Box 2728, Van Nuys, CA 91404.

Sky-Lab Foods, Incorporated, 4 Warehouse Lane, Elmsford, N.Y. 10523

Index

Page numbers in *italic* indicate illustrations or tables.